W9-BKU-213

LISA NEAL

feeding the bump

NUTRITION & RECIPES
FOR PREGNANCY

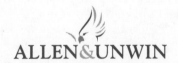

ALLEN&UNWIN

This book is intended as a source of information, not as a medical reference book. The reader is advised to consult with their medical health practitioner before, during and after their pregnancy and to inform their health professional about what food they are eating and any other regimes they are undertaking at all times.

While every care has been taken in compiling the information contained herein neither the author nor the publisher can be held responsible for any adverse reactions to the ingredients, recipes or suggestion offered and the use of any such information is entirely the reader's own decision.

Copyright © Lisa Neal 2008

All rights reserved. No part of this book may be reproduced or transmitted in any form or by any means, electronic or mechanical, including photocopying, recording or by any information storage and retrieval system, without prior permission in writing from the publisher. The *Australian Copyright Act 1968* (the Act) allows a maximum of one chapter or 10 per cent of this book, whichever is the greater, to be photocopied by any educational institution for its educational purposes provided that the educational institution (or body that administers it) has given a remuneration notice to Copyright Agency Limited (CAL) under the Act.

Allen & Unwin
83 Alexander Street
Crows Nest NSW 2065
Australia
Phone: (61 2) 8425 0100
Fax: (61 2) 9906 2218
Email: info@allenandunwin.com
Web: www.allenandunwin.com

National Library of Australia
Cataloguing-in-Publication entry:

Neal, Lisa, 1968– .
  Feeding the bump: nutrition & recipes for pregnancy.

  Bibliography.
  Includes index.
  ISBN: 9781741753714 (pbk.).

  1. Pregnancy – Nutritional aspects. 2. Lactation –
  Nutritional aspects. 3. Mothers – Nutrition. 4. Cookery.
  I. Title.

618.242

Patterns used throughout: *Indian Textile Prints*, The Peppin Press (www.peppinpress.com)
Typeset in 9.5/13.5 Minion by Midland Typesetters, Australia
Printed by McPherson's Printing Group, Australia.

10 9 8 7 6 5 4 3

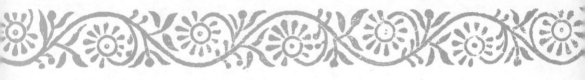

❁ contents

❀ Acknowledgements

Offering information on something as vital as diet during pregnancy bears incredible responsibility. For that reason this book is based on extensive research and interviews with the following professionals:

Professor Michael J. Bennett	Obstetrician, Royal Hospital for Women, Sydney
Kate di Prima	Dietitian and Spokesperson for Dietitians Association of Australia, Brisbane
Joy Heads	Head Lactation Consultant, Royal Hospital for Women, Sydney
Natasha Longhurst	Dietitian, Royal Prince Alfred Hospital, Sydney
Karen Redrup	Midwife, Royal Prince Alfred Hospital, Sydney
Catherine Major	Naturopath, Sydney

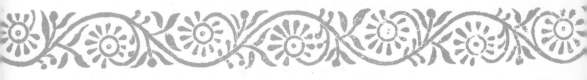

✿ Praise for Feeding the Bump

Increasingly we learn that we are what we eat and at no time is this more important than during pregnancy. This publication is aimed at women who plan to become pregnant or are already pregnant and who wish to assist Mother Nature in giving their babies the best possible start. The advice is sound and the recipes should not be beyond anyone who cares to follow them and produce wholesome and healthy dishes.

Lisa Neal has put a great deal of time and effort into this 'baby' of hers and every pregnant woman who follows her advice can be confident she will have done her best for her unborn child.

Professor Michael J. Bennett, MB ChB, ND (UCT) FCOG (SA), FRCOG, FRANZCOG, DDU

Michael Bennett is the Professor of Obstetrics and Gynaecology and Head of the School of Obstetrics and Gynaecology at the University of New South Wales. He is also the Clinical Director of Benign Gynaecology at the Royal Hospital for Women in Sydney and Chairman of the Senior Medical Staff Council.

I believe *Feeding the Bump* is an excellent resource for pregnant women or the couple planning to fall pregnant. It contains practical, up-to-date and easy-to-understand nutritional information that will guide you through the complete 40 weeks of pregnancy. The sections on morning sickness and danger foods to avoid throughout pregnancy are incredibly helpful. The recipes are healthy and pay particular attention to the specific needs of pregnancy.

I wish Lisa had published this while I was pregnant. It is a book that I will regularly recommend patients and friends purchase. An essential guide for those starting their family.

Kate Di Prima, Accredited Practising Dietitian

Kate Di Prima is a dietitian with 15 years experience in family nutrition. She has a Masters in Nutrition and Dietetics and has three private practice clinics in Brisbane.

Being a busy woman with limited cooking skills, I was concerned about providing myself and my baby with a nutritious diet throughout my pregnancy. *Feeding the Bump* has been an invaluable resource—it is filled with useful information and tips about diet during pregnancy as well as simple recipes that even I could not get wrong. The food is healthy, yet full of flavour, and I love that the recipes are quick to prepare, limiting my time spent in the kitchen.

With so many factors out of my control during this special time in my life, it was comforting to know I was providing a diet rich in the nutrients that would give my bub the best possible start.

Katrina Warren, TV Presenter and new mum

We really wanted meals that would satisfy my changing nutritional requirements and be yummy for both of us. And they had to be quick and easy to cook; neither of us had much energy for making dinner at the end of a long day of work. I was eating meat only occasionally and, as a result, I didn't have much confidence about how to cook meat dishes, but I definitely felt like I wanted to eat it while I was pregnant. We were particularly pleased when Lisa sent us the recipe for Beef and Avocado Pesto Pasta—completely delicious! It was the first time I had cooked rump steak, and it was satisfying to make such a wonderful meal the first time! All of the recipes we tried were very easy to make, and I felt I was getting a wide range of nutrients in every meal: more than I might have had with the meals I usually made. I definitely recommend these recipes to other pregnant women. I'm sure that eating well contributed to my amazing experience of pregnancy, and to the fabulous health of our baby daughter.

Christy Newman, Research Fellow and new mum

I got my hands on *Feeding the Bump* half-way through my pregnancy and wished I'd had it from the outset. I was rather petrified about not eating the right things and found most of the information out there confusing and conflicting. After reading this book I realised I had been excluding many yummy things—cooked mussels, tuna, salmon, oysters and even omelettes—from my diet unnecessarily. Now I have this fabulous 'one-stop-shop' filled with the right information about eating well, healthily and sensibly during pregnancy. And it has the best recipes—easy to follow with ingredients you'd find in your cupboard or fridge. My personal favourite was the Tuna Nicoise. The 'top tips' were most informative plus allocating the recipes to the relevant trimester was an absolute brainwave. I love the juices, soups, dips and meat dishes—in fact all of it—and so does my husband. Knowing that I am eating well for our baby is most reassuring and empowering.

Cathy Tropiano, expecting her first baby soon.

❀ Introduction

Feeding the Bump was conceived after an unsuccessful search for a cookbook to give as a gift to expecting parents. I was looking for a contemporary one that provided recipes rich in the nutrients specific to pregnancy. There was nothing available, which I found astounding considering the importance of diet and nutrition during this time, as did the many mothers I have since interviewed.

I have always believed that food is medicine. When applied to pregnancy I began to wonder whether diet could contribute to a more comfortable pregnancy. I also wondered whether you could coordinate eating foods rich in specific nutrients that are appropriate to specific stages of foetal growth and development. My aim was to optimise this development through diet. Research proves you can. Vitamins A and D are essential for eye development during the first trimester; and omega 3 is crucial during the third trimester for brain development. If 'you are what you eat', it is not a stretch to say 'your baby is what you eat'.

Diet is one of the most important factors in pregnancy. It is also the only factor you can have complete influence over. You can contribute towards a comfortable pregnancy and help grow a beautiful healthy baby simply by eating delicious, nutritious food. Studies show babies of well-nourished mothers are much healthier than babies born to mothers whose diets were lacking essential nutrients. Further evidence proves that good nutrition in pregnancy continues into childhood and adulthood, while undernourished babies are more susceptible to infection and disease throughout their lives.

Your developing baby relies on you for *all* of its nutritional needs. A balanced diet will ensure you are providing the best possible environment for your baby to grow and start life with the gift of good health. And the benefits are twofold. A healthy mum-to-be is more likely to have an enjoyable pregnancy. Diet can assist to minimise, or even avoid, many of the common complaints of pregnancy. Plus a healthy woman will recover more quickly from childbirth and find it easier to get back into shape; weight gained from healthy calories is much easier to lose. There is no need to change your diet radically or follow a restricted eating plan, you just need to be aware of the foods needed for a healthy pregnancy.

Ensuring your body is using the food you eat efficiently is another important factor. By combining certain foods you can maximise the absorption of your nutrients. For example, the absorption of iron is doubled when eaten with foods rich in vitamin C.

There are over 100 recipes in this book, all carefully devised to provide the right nutrients at the right time. To this end, the recipes are divided into three chapters representing the three trimesters of pregnancy. Each trimester has characteristic symptoms and discomforts, as well as its specific stages of foetal development. It makes perfect sense to plan your diet with foods that can manage these symptoms as well as maximise development.

As the baby grows and develops, its nutritional needs change. It relies on its mother for these needs. A mother has her own nutritional needs to meet *and* has to deal with the physical challenges that come with pregnancy. These issues are addressed by identifying at each trimester the:

- stage of foetal growth and development
- physical and dietary demands of the expecting mother
- symptoms and discomforts common to that trimester and food remedies to assist managing them.

These recipes deliver and meet each trimester's needs. There are recipes to assist with nausea in the first trimester and others are rich in iron to prevent anaemia in the second trimester—two common complaints of pregnancy. For the baby, we focus on calcium-rich meals during the second trimester as bones begin to harden. During the third trimester you will find recipes that boast omega 3 and iodine, required for optimum brain development.

Some nutritional needs are similar throughout pregnancy, such as protein, and so many recipes can be enjoyed at any time during your pregnancy to increase your choice. Recipes are clearly marked according to their nutritional content and benefits. You can use this as a guide in planning a healthy pregnancy diet suitable to your own tastes and needs.

Food aversions and fatigue are common during pregnancy and are not conducive to inspiring you to whip up a nutritionally balanced meal three times a day, let alone healthy snacks. Considering how important diet is during pregnancy it is best to be armed, so every recipe in this book is nutritionally loaded.

The recipes are easy to follow and many can be prepared in 30 minutes or less. There are meals that require a little more planning and a longer cooking time but they are still simple to follow and are well worth the effort. They can often also be the dishes that yield a few meal servings and so are time efficient overall. Readily available ingredients are used, with seasonal alternatives when appropriate. Some meals can be pre-cooked and frozen with an emphasis on convenient *on-the-go* snacks. You will find that snacks are essential to the pregnancy diet.

Feeding the Bump is based on extensive research and interviews with obstetricians, dietitians, naturopaths, midwives and mothers. It does not claim to be a medical authority but it does offer quick, simple recipes beneficial to a healthy pregnancy. It will allow you to become more aware of what to eat in order to meet your additional nutritional needs.

Diet is of course important during pregnancy but this doesn't mean food should not be enjoyed. The aim of *Feeding the Bump* is to relieve the anxiety of what, when and how to eat when expecting.

3

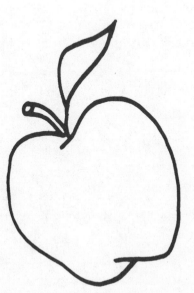

Part one

Food and Nutrition for Pregnancy

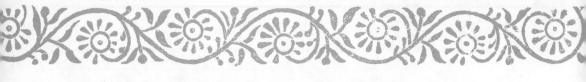

❀ The Importance of Diet During Pregnancy

Your baby is solely dependent upon you to supply all of the nutrients required for growth, energy and development. A nutrient deficiency obviously also has an affect on your own health. It can also compromise your ability to maintain the pregnancy and nourish your growing baby. Every aspect of your reproductive health, including the uterus, placenta and breast milk, is directly affected by what you eat. By eating well, you diminish these concerns.

Friends and colleagues often remark that women have been successfully delivering babies for thousands of years without folate supplements or dietary advice. This is true, but if you look back throughout history (and still today in some cultures) pregnant women were nurtured, protected and even restricted to bed, with pregnancy regarded as a very special phase of life. Today, women work in more high-profile jobs and choose to have children at a later age. We have more demanding and stressful lifestyles, access to an unlimited range of processed foods and, unless you are eating only organic foods, the fruits and vegetables available today are perhaps not as nutritionally rich as our ancestor's choices were. It is for all of these reasons that we need to place more focus on diet during pregnancy.

Your growing baby essentially eats the food you eat. Food is broken down, absorbed and distributed as energy and nutrients via the bloodstream. The placenta draws nourishment directly from your bloodstream and in turn nourishes the foetus. It will absorb everything that enters your body. This is why alcohol is a particular worry. The foetus absorbs alcohol from your bloodstream, but in a much more concentrated form. Compare your body mass to that of your unborn and you can understand the concern.

Dieting and skipping meals can also be dangerous. As blood sugar levels drop from lack of food, not only do you deny yourself energy, you also deprive your baby of the fuel it needs to grow and develop. A foetus never stops growing and needs this constant supply of energy. In fact, the best and most common advice given about planning a pregnancy diet is to eat small, regular meals, and you can prevent most of the complaints of pregnancy by doing so.

Try to eat every two to three hours, five to six times a day, and make breakfast the most important meal of your day. No one, pregnant or otherwise, should skip breakfast. It refuels your body after a fast and keeps blood sugar levels in check from the word go. If you find

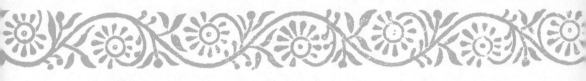

it difficult to eat in the morning, have a single slice of toast or a healthy smoothie until you can stomach something more substantial.

Studies carried out at Harvard School of Public Health have proven how much a newborn's health is a result of its mother's diet during pregnancy. Of the women in the study who had nutritionally balanced diets, 95 per cent gave birth to babies in excellent health. Only 8 per cent of women with poor nutritional diets gave birth to babies in good to excellent health.

Looking after yourself goes hand in hand with producing a healthy baby. Your body works harder during pregnancy than at any other time in your life. Your major organs function faster and more efficiently to cope with the increased blood supply required in pregnancy. Your heart works 40 per cent harder, pumping extra blood around your body. Your lungs keep this blood enriched with oxygen and your kidneys clean and filter it. A well-nourished diet ensures excellent health and strength of your organs and constantly replenishes essential nutrients. This is important because kidneys cannot distinguish between waste and nutrients. Water-soluble nutrients (vitamins C and B-group) are excreted and lost at a much higher rate when pregnant as the body flushes more fluids out more quickly.

The benefits of being healthy

Inadequate nutrition in the first trimester can impair your baby's development. Inadequate nutrition in the third trimester can hinder your baby's growth. Inadequate nutrition throughout the entire pregnancy can compromise immune function, leaving you vulnerable to infections. Well-nourished mothers, though, are more likely to produce babies of a correct birth weight and their babies are generally more mentally alert and have a stronger resistance to disease.

Many people claim they don't have time to be healthy, and with fad diets and conflicting information it can seem daunting and time-consuming to eat. It may seem a whole lot easier to take advantage of time-saving meal options, but this usually means highly processed choices.

The challenges of pregnancy—nausea, fatigue and food aversions—can make planning a wholesome meal totally undesirable. But you need to make sure that every meal you eat during your pregnancy will be the best choice for you and your baby, in fact the whole family. A healthy diet has many rewards. You will feel great and add longevity to your life, all the while knowing you are doing the best for your baby. Fresh food also tastes so much better than processed foods and if you follow a highly nutritious diet you can happily enjoy the occasional (and naughty) treat. We are, after all, only human. A healthy diet can:

- reduce a mother's risk of developing anaemia, pre-eclampsia, hypertension and long-term diseases, including diabetes and osteoporosis
- contribute to a more comfortable pregnancy by avoiding or minimising symptoms such as fatigue, nausea, constipation, leg cramps, reflux and heartburn
- help prepare for labour and delivery—energy stores help you endure labour, while a healthy uterus can 'push' more effectively and well-nourished women are less likely to deliver early
- stabilise your emotional state—a balanced diet helps moderate mood swings and anxiety
- lend towards a quicker recovery—a healthy body seems to bounce back faster, with an easier return to pre-pregnancy body weight
- ensure nutritional breast milk for a happy, healthy baby
- provide you with more energy to enjoy your newborn—a quick recovery leaves you less fatigued and less likely to suffer postnatal depression.

A well-nourished woman is also more likely to experience a more comfortable pregnancy. There are discomforts or symptoms common to being pregnant namely morning sickness, fatigue, digestive problems, constipation and stretch marks. And there are the more serious conditions of hypertension, anaemia, gestational diabetes and pre-eclampsia. The good news is that all of these conditions can be relieved, and even avoided, by good diet.

Food is medicine. It's a natural remedy that encourages your body to cure and heal itself while building up resistance to infection and disease. Food remedies have been curing illness and ailments for centuries. But the proof is in the pudding. I practice this philosophy in my life and I can't remember the last time I took any form of prescriptive medicine and I rarely get sick. Eating fabulous food keeps me healthy.

A nourishing diet is the best form of preventative medicine. This is especially relevant when pregnant as it is generally not recommended to take medication while expecting, not even a cold and flu tablet! So it is easy to conclude that a well-balanced diet is your best bet for a healthy and happy pregnancy.

A weighty matter

Many obstetricians and midwives do not like to place too much emphasis or importance on a specific weight gain for each trimester. Some practitioners even choose not to weigh their patients, unless there are signs of extreme weight loss or gain. They will, though, still monitor your weight, if not by scales then by sight, to ensure you are progressing within the healthy range.

Most women will gain between 9 to 13 kilograms (19 to 28 pounds)—more for twins—during their pregnancy. Most of this weight is attributed to the placenta, increased blood supply, fat stores for lactation and an expanded uterus to support the growing baby.

Gradual weight gain will ensure your baby will grow steadily and be born at a healthy birth weight. It will also ensure you have more control over the more serious conditions of pregnancy (diabetes, hypertension and pre-eclampsia), and help you to return to your pre-pregnancy weight more easily.

Controlled weight gain can reduce the risk of complications that may arise from being either too under- or overweight. Concerns related to underweight women include:

- trouble conceiving
- higher risk of premature delivery and low birth weight babies, who can be more susceptible to disease and infection throughout their life
- high metabolism of protein and fat stores make up for lack of energy and this process can produce toxins known as ketones that are hazardous to the foetus
- inadequate breast milk as fat stores are essential to breastfeeding.

Concerns related to overweight women include:
- larger babies that can lead to difficult childbirths and higher incidence of stitches, tears and wound infections for the mother
- high risk of developing pelvic inflammation due to excess weight and pressure on the uterus
- diabetes
- varicose veins and stretch marks
- haemorrhoids
- high blood pressure and pre-eclampsia
- backaches and leg cramps
- additional stress and strain on skeleton and all organs (especially heart and kidneys)
- low energy levels.

Not much weight is generally gained during the first trimester, maybe 1 to 2 kilograms. Food intake should not need to increase too much in the first months, unless you have been professionally advised to or your appetite indicates otherwise. The body is very clever in making known its needs, so listen to it and (sensibly) feed it what it needs.

As your pregnancy progresses, so does your need for extra energy. The third trimester sees the most weight gained, with a rapidly growing baby triggering an increase in appetite. On average an extra 600 kilojoules are needed per day towards the end of pregnancy. This is easily achieved by adding one of the following to your daily intake:

- an extra glass of milk
- 2 slices of cheese
- 1 x 200 g/7 oz tub of yoghurt
- 2 slices of bread
- 2 pieces of fruit
- 2 slices of lean meat.

Your body will only demand what it needs to meet extra energy needs. Nutritional requirements however, double, so you need to meet this quota without doubling food intake. Every mouthful counts. Every recipe—even snacks and drinks—need to be loaded with nutritional goodness.

While a moderately low-fat diet should be followed, pregnant women should never follow a restricted calorie diet. Dieting denies the baby adequate energy for proper growth and development. By eliminating 'good' fats from your diet, you limit the essential fatty acids that are vital to a healthy pregnancy.

Do not miss a meal. And never fast during pregnancy. You are simply starving your baby by doing so. Inadequate calories can increase the risk of miscarriage and premature delivery. It can promote abnormalities and slow foetal growth. Skipping meals causes blood sugar levels to drop and that can trigger nausea, fatigue and put you at high risk of developing gestational diabetes. Eat regularly, every two to three hours, *before* you get hungry.

Low GI foods

The recipes in this book are based on the low GI philosophy. The glycaemic index (GI) is a measurement of the rate at which sugar enters the bloodstream. Low GI foods are recommended in a healthy diet as they are foods that are digested well and release energy at a slow and steady rate. This helps to control blood sugar levels and diabetes. It also helps to satisfy the appetite for longer periods.

High GI foods are digested quickly and cause blood glucose levels to rise and then fall rapidly. This can result in an energy slump or fatigue. On rare occasions, high GI foods can play a role in the pregnancy diet. Blood pressure or blood sugar can unexpectedly drop, making you feel dizzy or faint. A natural sugar fix—fresh or dried fruit—can ease these symptoms immediately.

Including low GI foods in the diet also helps to prevent diabetes, obesity and heart disease and lower blood fats and sustain energy levels. Low GI food choices include most of the foods already recommended for pregnancy, such as:

- unrefined wholegrain products—oats, buckwheat, barley, sourdough bread and dense breads with visible grains. It is important to note that wholemeal bread has a high GI count as opposed to wholegrain, which is low
- durum wheat pasta, basmati rice and doongara rice
- all legumes, including lentils and chickpeas
- low-fat milk, soy milk and yoghurt
- all non-starchy vegetables, including dark green leafy vegetables, cauliflower, celery, leeks, mushrooms and sweet potato
- apples, bananas, berries, pears, prunes, kiwi fruit, mangoes, stone fruit (especially apricots) and oranges.

11

✿ foods to Avoid

An expectant mother is bombarded with countless contradicting claims about what she should and should not do, especially regarding diet. However, obstetricians, dietitians and government health organisations do agree about what foods should be avoided, or minimised from your diet during pregnancy.

- You must avoid: raw fish, uncooked meats, organ meats and soft, unpasteurised and imported cheeses.
- You need to minimise: sugar, alcohol, caffeine and processed or refined foods that contain chemicals and preservatives.

fish

Fish is an excellent source of nutrition. It is rich in protein, zinc, iodine, omega 3, vitamins B12 and D and many minerals and is very low in saturated fat. It is important to make it a regular, essential part of the pregnancy diet. Having said that, there has been a lot of concern about the effect of high mercury levels found in fish.

A foetus is much more susceptible to the toxic effect of mercury than an adult. It can affect the development of the baby's central nervous system and cause kidney damage. Fish species at the top of the food chain, such as shark, swordfish and fresh tuna fillets, do usually contain higher mercury levels. These species should either be avoided or eaten minimally. To be safe, Food Standards Australia New Zealand make the following dietary recommendations:

> 1 serve per fortnight of shark, broadbill, swordfish, marlin, fresh tuna (and no other fish that fortnight)
>
> OR 1 serve per week of deep sea perch (orange roughy) or catfish and no other fish that week
>
> OR 2 to 3 servings per week of any fish or seafood not listed above.

There are many seafood recipes to choose from in this book, using fish species with low recorded mercury levels. You can therefore enjoy all the benefits of eating seafood up to three times a week! The following fish are high in omega 3 and low in mercury levels: Atlantic salmon, canned salmon and tuna, sardines (fresh and canned), mackerel, silver warehou, snapper and trevally.

Canned fish is an excellent and convenient source of fish and canned tuna is safe to eat during pregnancy. The smaller species of tuna generally used for canning have much lower levels of mercury than fresh tuna steaks. Food Standards Australia New Zealand has calculated that is it safe to consume 95 grams (3½ ounces) canned tuna every day when no other fish is eaten.

Shellfish must always be cooked when eaten during pregnancy. Mussels are a fantastic source of the essential mineral zinc, so cook and enjoy. Always ensure you purchase your seafood fresh and from reputable suppliers.

> The nutrient selenium is thought to protect the body against heavy-metal poisoning such as mercury. Food rich sources are brazil nuts, chicken, garlic, mushrooms and . . . seafood. If you are concerned about your mercury levels, include more of these foods in your diet.

❀ Healthy food Preparation and hygiene

- Wash your hands with soap before preparing food and between touching raw meats and cooked food.

- Thoroughly wash and dry raw fruit and vegetables, removing all traces of soil prior to use.

- Thaw frozen foods in the refrigerator, not at room temperature. Bacteria thrive at room temperature.

- Keep food hot or cold. Do not leave food at room temperature for more than 30 minutes.

- Store raw meat separately from all other foods and thoroughly wash utensils used in preparation.

- Thorough cooking destroys listeria. Ensure all food is cooked through—this includes all red and white meats and fish, which must be cooked until flesh turns opaque. Hold the medium/rare requests for now.

- Re-heat food until steaming hot throughout.

- Do not re-freeze food once thawed.

- Aim to eat freshly cooked food. When eating out, try to avoid smorgasbords and salad bars.

- Do not eat any food if there is any doubt about its hygienic preparation or storage.

- Discard food with any sign of ageing or mould. Cutting off a contaminated section is not enough as bacteria may have penetrated the whole food.

- Keep your refrigerator clean. Wipe spills and keep temperature below 5°C/40°F.

- Do not cut or prepare raw meat on wooden chopping boards. Wash all boards in hot soapy water after use.

- Avoid any foods that are past their 'best before' or 'use by' date, especially refrigerated foods.

- Listeria survives and grows in the fridge, so contaminated foods must be destroyed.

uncookeD anD oRgan meats

Raw (including cure meats, such as Parma ham), rare and undercooked meat or poultry of any kind may contain salmonella bacteria and the toxoplamosis parasite. Needless to say, these should be avoided. If you come into contact with toxoplasmosis during your first trimester it can be harmful to the foetus as it can cross the placenta. Listeria is also another problem found with these meats.

Liver and kidneys need to be avoided during pregnancy. They have very high concentrated levels of vitamin A which, like the supplements, can affect your baby's development. Vitamin A sourced from plant products in the form of beta-carotene is safe as the body will only convert what it needs.

Listeria

Listeria is bacteria found in sheep, cattle and other animals. It can cause food poisoning and is most commonly contracted via unpasteurised, unrefrigerated or contaminated food products, such as undercooked meat, raw fish and soft cheeses. It is not usually life-threatening if contracted by an adult, but it can pose serious problems for the developing baby, resulting in miscarriage, premature birth or, in the most extreme cases, stillbirth. Symptoms of listeriosis may include fever, headache, tiredness and aches and pains. High-risk foods for listeria include:

- raw fish and chilled seafood—sushi and ready-to-eat peeled prawns
- undercooked meat—beef, lamb, pork and chicken
- cold cooked meats—chicken, ham
- soft cheeses—brie, camembert, blue cheese, feta and ricotta (can be eaten if cooked until steaming)
- pressed meats, salami, pate, uncooked smoked fish, olives sold in open deli counters (bottled or canned olives are safe)
- soft serve ice-cream.

Listeria can be easily avoided by making careful food choices and following hygienic food preparation and storage. This practice should be carried out whether pregnant or not. Listeria is killed by pasteurisation and any unpasteurised, soft mouldy cheese or any cheese that sits in water is a high-risk food. Imported cheeses are generally unpasteurised. Hard (pasteurised) cheeses are perfectly safe choices. It is imperative to check 'use by' dates on perishable dairy products prior to eating. Safe dairy choices include:

- hard cheese—parmesan, cheddar and edam cheese
- soft cheese—cream and cottage cheese (eat within 24 hours of opening sealed packaging)
- yoghurt and pasteurised milk.

Sugar

Refined sugar contains no nutritional value, whether raw, white or brown. It provides wasted calories that can be replaced easily with delicious nourishing options. Sugar puts a lot of strain on your body's digestive system and hormone production (insulin) making it difficult to maintain normal blood sugar levels. Blood sugar levels need to be controlled in order to avoid the onset of gestational diabetes, high blood pressure, dizziness, fainting, nausea and fatigue. Your body works hard and uses more energy to control sugar when it enters the bloodstream. This explains the slump usually experienced after high sugar consumption. Sugar also increases your need for zinc and B group vitamins (especially folate) and can interfere with the absorption of calcium. These are all-important nutrients during pregnancy.

Sugar cravings can indicate a lack of complex carbohydrates in the diet. In fact, complex carbohydrates are an effective way of controlling sugar cravings. If you have a sweet tooth, sweeten your desserts or baked goods naturally and nutritiously with dried fruits such as apricots, prunes and raisins, or fresh apple, pear or orange juice. As fruit is high in natural sugars it also needs to be consumed in reasonable moderation. Experts suggest eating three to four servings of fruit a day.

Replacing sugar with artificial sweeteners is not recommended. They are made with chemicals and are toxic, especially to the liver. Honey is a more natural option and if a recipe calls for sweetening I will always take the natural way. Honey has a lower GI rating than sugar and has antibacterial, antioxidant and medicinal properties. New Zealand manuka honey is especially good. Honey is still a concentrated form of sugar, though, so aim to keep intake to a minimum.

Sugar is added to most of the processed and packaged food available today. Reading food labels before you buy is the best way to keep tabs on what you are really eating. Avoid anything with 'added' sugar, which comes under many disguises of glucose, sucrose or dextrose. Tinned fruit in syrup, sweetened cereals and health food bars are sneaky suspects.

Of course at some stage we all give into the occasional sugar fix but if you follow a healthy and nutrient-rich diet the odd indulgence is not going to jeopardise your health. A handy tip is to combine your sugar hit with fibre. Fibre controls the rate at which sugar is absorbed into the bloodstream, which can help to control the blood sugar peak.

15

Add cocoa for chocolate high-fibre muffins, or eat a small portion of dark chocolate after a meal containing lentils or vegetables.

Obviously I am not suggesting you devour an entire bar of chocolate after each and every fibre-rich meal. Sensible eating is always the key to good health and I am sure you will enjoy the delicious variety of healthy desserts in this book. Chances are, you won't even notice the absence of refined sugar in your diet.

> Dark chocolate and good quality cocoa are the best choices for chocoholics. Both are rich in iron and high in antioxidants.

Caffeine

Caffeine and tannic acid found in tea and coffee can inhibit the absorption of iron, so it is best to avoid drinking them with a meal. It also acts as a diuretic and can deplete you and your baby of essential fluids. Always replenish these lost fluids with water.

Studies are underway regarding other concerns about the effects of caffeine on the developing baby, but generally health authorities recommend discontinuing or reducing caffeine consumption during pregnancy. Ask your health practitioner to suggest beneficial herbal teas to drink as a substitute.

Alcohol

The National Health and Medical Research Council recommends that if you are planning to become pregnant or if you are pregnant then you need to consider not drinking alcohol at all. Most importantly, you should never become intoxicated. The risk from alcohol to your baby is thought to be higher during the early stages of pregnancy, from conception to the first missed period. Alcohol passes through the placenta and it is difficult to identify the exact levels that may cause harm. Most professionals advise you to consider not drinking alcohol at all.

Processed and refined foods

These should be minimised in any diet, not just during pregnancy. They are nutritionally depleted, wasted calories and generally have hidden additives that put undue stress on the body and its digestive system.

Today we have access to a huge range of fresh, healthy food with organic options becoming more and more accessible and affordable. Besides, natural food always tastes so much better. What can compare to a ripe, juicy mango, fresh hot bread or a succulent salmon fillet straight from the oven?

❀ Tips for healthy cooking

- Eat fruit and vegetables raw whenever possible.

- Choose lean cuts of meat and chicken and trim off visible fat before cooking.

- Bake, steam or grill rather than fry. These methods require little or no fat to cook. Baking allows for a more even cooking temperature, with little or no loss of water-soluble vitamins. Dry bake vegetables on baking paper for a deliciously low-fat alternative, or bake whole fruits such as apples, peaches or plums for a simple, healthy dessert. Steaming is preferred to boiling as fewer nutrients leach out into the water.

- Stir-fry in chicken stock rather than oil.

- Use non-stick frying pans—a great investment towards good health.

- Keep cooking time to a minimum and do not overcook foods as you will compromise on flavour and goodness.

- Cook from scratch—it is rewarding and you know exactly what you are eating.

- Store foods in a dark, cool place as nutritional loss is accelerated by light and heat.

- Prepare fruits and vegetables just prior to eating as peeling and cutting activates nutritional loss, especially in vitamin C sources.

- Marinate to tenderise meats as it reduces cooking time and loss of nutrients. Use fresh herbs and spices to add flavour as well as nutrition—they decrease the need for fats and processed sauces.

- Use avocado as a spread or toss through steamed vegetables rather than butter—it is food for your baby's brain and your skin will love you for it.

- Bake with buttermilk as it is a low-fat dairy product similar to but not as thick and tart as yoghurt.

- Incorporate skim milk powder into recipes—it is a fabulous source of calcium and protein. Add to smoothies, soups and baked goods.

- Substitute toasted wheatgerm for breadcrumbs in crumbles and toppings for a massive nutritional boost.

- Opt for tomato rather than cream- or butter-based sauces.

- Avoid adding salt to foods. Flavour with herbs and spices or dried seaweed. Seaweed is high in iodine and zinc and available from health food stores.

🏵 HOW TO fill a Pregnant Belly

A balanced diet is the key to good health. High quality protein, loads of fresh vegetables, fruit, calcium-rich foods and small amounts of unsaturated fats should be included in your daily diet. Being aware of the essential nutrients that are important to a healthy pregnancy is a key factor in planning this.

Our bodies require seven nutrients, vital to good health, proper growth and to carry out all of our bodily functions. These include carbohydrates, protein, fibre, vitamins and minerals, fats and water. A balance of these foods must be consumed each and every day.

It sounds daunting but don't despair—all recipes in this book have been carefully planned and devised to maximise the full nutritional benefits of food.

CarbohyDrates 8 servings Daily

Carbohydrates are an important energy source for an expecting mother. They are also the baby's main source of energy from which to grow and develop. Carbohydrates feed the brain, they help form protein and fight toxins. They break down to form glucose which fuels our muscles and controls blood sugar levels.

There are two types of carbohydrates: simple carbohydrates and complex carbohydrates.

Simple carbohydrates: include fruit (fresh and dried). They provide a quick but short-lasting burst of energy. This boosts blood sugar levels so they must be eaten in moderation. While fruit is definitely a much healthier option than cakes or sweets, it is advised to eat no more than three to four pieces a day. It seems crazy to have to limit such healthy foods, but it is more important to control blood sugar levels during pregnancy. Select fruits with a low GI count, such as apples, apricots, pears, berries, kiwi fruit, citrus fruits, mangoes and firm bananas (ripe bananas have a higher GI rating). One serving size for smaller fruits, such as apricots and kiwi fruit, equals two pieces of fruit.

Complex carbohydrates: provide a more stable and slower release of energy to the body. This satisfies the appetite quicker and for longer. Complex carbohydrates are usually rich in vitamins and minerals and high in dietary fibre (essential for avoiding constipation).

Best food sources include: wholegrains and their products—bread, cereals, brown rice and pasta—legumes and lentils, vegetables, seeds and nuts.

Eight to ten servings a day of low GI-rated carbohydrates are recommended during pregnancy. One serving equals 30 grams (1 ounce) or in food terms, any of the following: 2 slices of bread; 2 pieces of fruit; 4 crackers; 1 cup of cooked rice; 1 cup of cooked pasta; 1 cup of cereal or 1 medium potato.

In view of the low-carb/no carb fads of recent years, note that restricting carbohydrates during pregnancy can actually be dangerous and retard foetal growth. Glucose is the primary source of energy used to develop the baby's nervous system.

Aim to avoid refined carbohydrates such as white bread, rice and pasta, cakes, biscuits and processed cereals. They are nutritionally inferior to their wholegrain partners and generally contain less fibre. High fibre breads might have *high fibre*, but they still do not have all the nutrients found in wholegrain products. Don't be fooled by claims these products are '*enriched with added nutrients*'. They really should not have been taken out in the first place.

Protein   3 to 4 servings Daily

Protein is found in every cell of our body. It builds muscles, bones, skin and organs. It supports the immune system, repairs the body, promotes muscle responses and is a valuable source of energy. Protein is needed for healthy blood and to transport oxygen around the body. It also aids digestion by releasing enzymes to satisfy the appetite—one of many reasons why protein should be included in every meal.

Protein is very important. For the mother, it is needed for the production of blood cells to support the extra blood required during pregnancy. It maintains healthy breasts, and the uterus and muscle strength required in labour. Healthy levels of protein are useful in controlling fatigue and anaemia. For the baby, protein forms the structure of every growing tissue and cell. It builds and nourishes bones, muscles, skin and all vital organs.

It is important to get your protein intake right. Research shows that inadequate protein levels can lead to low birth weight or smaller babies. A lack of protein in the third trimester can also interfere with brain development. However, high protein diets are *not* recommended for pregnant women. When proteins are digested they produce a chemical that in excess can be harmful to the foetus. Too much protein can also cause or aggravate constipation and haemorrhoids. As with all foods, eat in moderation, although high-protein supplement shakes should definitely be avoided.

High quality protein food sources should be included in all meals from the beginning of your pregnancy, with intake increasing moderately during the third trimester. The amount of protein to eat varies, depending upon the sources (animal or plant) and your level of

19

activity. Highly active mums need to double their intake, while those who are less active need only slightly increase theirs. Generally speaking, the daily intake of protein during pregnancy is approximately 50 grams/2 ounces. This is eaten over three to four servings that contain 15 grams/½ ounce of protein per serve. Examples of one serve include 2 eggs, or 60 grams/2½ ounces meat, chicken or fish, or 1 cup of baked beans. It is recommended you discuss your individual protein needs with your health practitioner, especially if protein intake was low at the time of, or prior to, conceiving.

Your diet should consist of first-class proteins that are low in saturated fat and kinder to your hearts. Believe it or not, hardening of the arteries (atherosclerosis) can even begin in toddlers. Select lean red meat, skinless chicken and turkey, and low-fat dairy products. Fish is a fabulous low-fat source of protein and is an essential part of the pregnancy diet. Nuts are a fantastic source of plant protein. They are high in fat but contain the 'good' unsaturated fats needed to sustain a normal and healthy pregnancy. Even so, eat in moderation.

Proteins are also divided into two groups: animal and vegetable proteins.

Animal proteins are a complete protein. This means they contain the nine essential amino acids (building blocks) required by the body. They also tend to be high in saturated fat.

Best food sources include: lean red meat, poultry (skinless chicken and turkey, pork in moderation), seafood (always cooked), eggs, low-fat dairy products, hard cheese.

Vegetable proteins are usually lower in fat but do not individually contain all nine essential amino acids. Tofu is an exception to this rule, making it the only non-animal complete protein. New studies are advising that tofu and its products should not be eaten in excess, so vegetarians are advised not to rely solely on tofu for their protein. Like any food and like any diet, variety and moderation are the keys to good health. Enjoy two to three servings per week to reap the nutritional benefits of this food.

Best food sources include: legumes (chickpeas, cannellini beans, black eyed peas, lentils), soy products (tofu, soy milk and soy cheese), wholegrains (wheatgerm and quinoa, buckwheat, wholegrain bread and cereals), nuts and seeds.

Vegetarian mothers need to be particularly aware of their protein intake. More servings and variety are usually required to ensure all of the essential amino acids are consumed over the course of a day. Vary your protein choices in each meal and be aware of the beneficial food combinations. By combining vegetable proteins correctly you can achieve the same nutritional value as eating red meat. Vegetarian mothers also need to monitor their intake of iron, B12 and calcium. Again, these nutrients are all best absorbed by the body from animal sources.

Vegans should pay special attention to their diet and food sources, with greater quantities needed than the suggested animal sources. Protein will need to come from a variety of soy products, pulses and nuts. Calcium can be obtained from soy products (enriched with calcium), nuts and seeds (almonds are the richest source) and dark green vegetables (especially broccoli). Iron should be sourced from a combination of dark green vegetables, nuts, pulses and wholegrains. Consume these with foods rich in vitamin C to maximise absorption. And vitamin B12 must be sourced from fortified breakfast cereals, soy products and brewers yeast.

fibre

A diet high in fibre is imperative during pregnancy. Dietary fibre, or roughage, promotes the function and regularity of the gastro-intestinal system. This is necessary to remove solid wastes and toxins from the body. A diet lacking in fibre-rich foods can result in constipation, a condition that is already exacerbated during pregnancy due to hormonal changes.

Best food sources include: wholegrains, legumes, fresh vegetables generally, fresh and dried fruit, preferably raw, most nuts and seeds.

It is best to avoid large amounts of 'processed bran' as it can move foods through the body too quickly. This does not allow the body time to completely break down the food or absorb all its goodness.

21

vitamins and minerals

Vitamins are vital to growth, development, the functioning of all organs and general good health. They help to break down and release energy from food, promote healthy skin and hair and help the body to use other nutrients efficiently, for example vitamin D for calcium, vitamin C for iron. Fresh fruit and vegetables are your best sources of vitamins. But vitamins are very easily lost during storage and cooking, particularly vitamin C and the B-group. For this reason it is best to eat foods as fresh as possible to obtain maximum nutrition.

Minerals are imperative for human life. Iron, zinc, calcium and iodine are known as essential trace minerals. They are needed for growth, building strong bones, nails, teeth and muscles. They assist in the formation of blood cells, the health of the nervous system, the production of hormones and the breakdown of nutrients. Minerals are found in some form or other in most whole foods.

Vitamins and minerals work best together in their natural state. They work in synergy, each playing a role in each other's functions. They cannot, and do not, work effectively alone. To achieve a healthy nutritional balance, your best sources are from a variety of fresh, wholesome foods. There is no substitute or supplement for mother nature.

✿ Tips for healthy eating

1. **Eat a well-balanced diet.** Make fresh, simple choices from the main food groups—eat a variety of proteins, carbohydrates, vitamins and minerals, healthy fats and water.

2. **Eat foods in or as close to their natural wholesome state as possible.** The less food is tampered with the more goodness it will retain, meaning you gain maximum nutrition from what you eat. Whole foods also contain the correct mix of enzymes for breakdown and absorption.

3. **Fresh is best.** Avoid processed foods whenever possible. Nutritional content is depleted during processing and these foods often contain hidden additives and preservatives, putting a greater demand on your digestive system. Stick to unrefined and fresh produce.

4. **Invest in good quality produce.** You will taste the difference and find little or no need to add salt, sugar or fat for flavour.

5. **Eat and buy foods in season, when they are at their nutritional peak and much cheaper.** Supermarkets stock most produce year round. A reliable indicator for seasonal produce can be price; it generally drops during peak season. Use this rule for fresh fruit and vegetables as well as for meat and fish. Enjoy lamb during springtime and ask your fishmonger what fish species are in season and at their best before purchasing.

6. **Eat a wide variety of foods.** Experts claim eating 37 different types of food per day will ensure a complete balance of all the essential nutrients. It sounds a lot, but you might be surprised at how many you already eat. Here are some ways this can be done:

   - *Mix up the grains.* Don't have bread with every meal. Choose from rice, pasta, legumes, oats and barley, or a combination of grains in natural muesli. These all contain less salt than bread. If you just can't live without your daily bread, vary your choices—mixed grain, rye, spelt, pita and flatbreads.
   - *Veg out.* There are endless choices available today. Enjoy a mix of green, yellow and red vegetables every day, both raw and cooked. Stir-fries and salads are a great way to achieve this.
   - *Get fruity.* Be more adventurous than the apple, orange or banana. Fruit salads are the perfect way to eat fruit.
   - *Go for colour.* This is nature's way of ensuring you make the best nutritional choices. Deep, rich, naturally coloured foods are often the most nutritious. Rich, red tomatoes boast loads of vitamin C. The darker the meat the higher

the level of iron. Beef and lamb have more iron per gram than chicken or fish. Include fruits and vegetables of every colour on your plate at every meal.

7. **Fuel your body wisely.** It is important to make nutritionally wise choices, such as low GI foods.

8. **Get the full nutritional benefits from your food.** Food must be broken down and digested before your body can absorb its goodness. To do this you need the correct balance of enzymes and digestive aids. These are found in vitamins and minerals and are best sourced from food rather than supplements.

9. **Avoid losing nutrients in food.** Water-soluble vitamins (C and B group, especially folate) can be lost during transit, storage and cooking. So:
   - eat foods raw whenever possible
   - make fresh choices when buying ingredients—avoid vegetables with limp or rubbery leaves, blemishes on fruit (can indicate bacteria), and select fish with shiny scales and clear eyes
   - do not wash or cut fruit and vegetables to store them—wash thoroughly just *prior* to use and prepare as close to serving time as possible
   - eat the most nutritionally perishable foods of your weekly shopping first—fish, chicken and then red meat; leafy greens such as spinach and broccoli, then fruit, including tomatoes, followed by root vegetables such as potatoes and carrots
   - use minimal water when cooking—steam, grill or bake.

10. **Read the labels.** Many foods are not what they seem. Sugar, salt and chemicals and preservatives are hidden in more foods than you would probably imagine. Even health foods such as dried fruit can be laced with preservative 220 (sulphur dioxide) to maintain shelf-life. Don't be fooled by manufacturers' appealing claims. Canned foods are a particular concern, especially canned fish, tomatoes, legumes and cooking stock. These usually contain high levels of salt (under the disguise of sodium). Opt for salt-reduced or no added salt brands. 'All natural' or 'No preservatives' statements do not ensure you are purchasing a healthy product. Sugar and salt are natural products and can be disguised under many names. The term 'light' can mean light on flavour rather than calories, e.g. olive oil. And 'low fat' may just be lower than its high-fat competitors, or contain more sugar for taste as in yoghurt. Ingredients must be listed in order of their proportion in the product, beginning with the highest. If honey, glucose or sucrose tops the list of your breakfast cereal, you are starting the day with an unhealthy bowl of sugar.

fats

Fats are essential to life. The body needs them for growth and repairs, to regulate body temperature, maintain insulin levels, for healthy eyes and skin and to cushion vital organs. They help lower cholesterol and prevent heart disease and cancer. Fats also support the unborn baby as it grows, are necessary for lactation and milk supply and are an effective remedy for constipation as they keep the bowels well-lubricated. In pregnancy, fats, especially those rich in the essential fatty acids, are necessary for:

- reproduction (problems in fertility or irregular or no menstrual cycle can occur if fat stores are too low)
- production of pregnancy hormones
- formation of collagen for skin elasticity
- development of baby's brain and eyes (especially in the third trimester and during lactation)
- the immune systems of both mother and baby
- the growth of the placenta.

There are two types of fats: unsaturated and saturated.

Unsaturated or vegetable fats—more affectionately called the 'good fats'—are a concentrated source of energy and contain essential fatty acids, omega 3 and vitamins A, E and K. These are all necessary for foetal development and it has even been suggested they may help lessen the risk of pre-term births.

Essential fatty acids are found in the wall of every cell of the human body. They cannot be produced by the body and so must be supplied by the diet. Essential fatty acids are best sourced from unsaturated fats.

Omega 3 is increasingly being recognised for its numerous health benefits. It is great food for the brain and therefore vital during the third trimester. In fact, as the brain is not fully developed at birth, omega 3 (and iodine) are an important part of the mother's diet during breastfeeding and the infant's diet for the first two years of its life.

Best food sources include: oily fish, such as salmon and sardines; avocados; hazelnuts, walnuts, pumpkin seeds and sunflower seeds; extra-virgin olive oil, canola, sunflower and grapeseed oil.

Saturated or animal fats, the 'bad fats', are mostly solid at room temperature and should be avoided as much as possible in any diet. Sources include butter, cheese and white fat on meats.

While fats are essential throughout pregnancy and into breastfeeding, make wise choices in the fats you eat. Fats do not need to be fatty to provide nutritional value. Lean cuts of meat are an adequate source.

> Extra-virgin olive oil goes through minimal processing, making it one of the best oils to consume for good health.

Nutrients for two

When seeking advice on your pregnancy diet, you will be clearly instructed not to 'eat for two' but to 'eat the nutrients for two'. While the former seems very appealing, doubling the nutrients seems downright daunting.

The pregnancy diet should be basically a healthy balanced one, but there are some key nutrients to focus on, with intake increasing between 30 to 100 per cent during pregnancy. These include folate (folic acid), iron, zinc, calcium and magnesium, b-group vitamins (especially B6 and B12), vitamin C, iodine and essential fatty acids (omega 3).

Folate (or folic acid)

Folate is crucial for the development of the central nervous system, the brain, the spine and overall healthy growth. The main focus on folate in pregnancy is that it drastically reduces the risk of neural tube defects (or spina bifida) by up to 70 per cent. Development of the neural tube occurs in the first month following conception, after which time the neural tube closes. If folate levels are low or insufficient during this very short period, the tube will fail to close properly and birth abnormalities may result.

The recommended daily allowance of folate doubles to 800 micrograms before and during pregnancy. This intake is crucial during the first six weeks after conception and, if you have the opportunity, up to four months prior to conception. Considering the risks at stake many women prefer, or are professionally advised, to take folic acid supplements. It is still important to sustain a diet high in natural folate-rich food sources. Discuss this with your health practitioner.

Folate is best absorbed when eaten with foods rich in vitamin B12. This can be as easy as eating leafy green vegetables with a steak. The two vitamins work in conjunction with one another to perform the vital tasks of producing red blood cells and forming DNA, which passes on genetic information from parents to baby. Note that alcohol and cigarettes interfere with the absorption of many nutrients, but especially folate.

The body cannot store folate and during pregnancy your body excretes four to five times its normal amount. Daily intake is imperative.

Best food sources include: green leafy vegetables (spinach, rocket, broccoli, asparagus and avocados), fruits (including papaya, oranges, bananas, berries, apricots and melons), wholegrain products, nuts and seeds, legumes and pulses.

As folate is a water-soluble vitamin, it is very easily lost in storage and cooking, especially at high temperatures, in microwaves and in large amounts of water. Your leafy greens should be eaten as fresh and as soon after purchase as possible and lightly cooked, if at all.

Meals rich in folate have obviously been a main focus of the recipes for the first trimester, but you will find these folate-rich foods continue to appear in all the recipes. Studies are proving that folate is beneficial for the full term of the pregnancy for complete and proper development of the neural spine.

Zinc

Zinc is said to be one of the most important minerals in pregnancy. It is necessary for the fertility of both men and women and without it reproduction will not occur. Zinc is found in every human body cell. It is needed for growth, brain and nerve formation, healing of wounds and healthy skin and hair. It is vital to many bodily functions, including digestion, metabolism and breathing. It also boosts the immune system.

During pregnancy, zinc assists in the development of all the baby's organs, skeleton, brains, eyes and the nervous and immune systems. It is excellent for the health of the mother's uterus. It tones and strengthens it in preparation for labour and can promote a quicker internal recovery after birth. It is also involved in the production of collagen. Collagen maintains the skin's elasticity, allowing it to stretch easily with your growing belly and reducing the likelihood of stretch marks.

Zinc deficiency is very common and usually the main cause of infertility. A lack of zinc during pregnancy can inhibit foetal growth and promote low birth weight babies. Zinc should therefore play a major role in the diet prior to and during the entire pregnancy. In fact it is important throughout our entire lives. Healthy levels of zinc during the third trimester have been linked to preventing premature births and postnatal depression.

Zinc is best absorbed from animal sources, so again vegetarians need to be conscious of their options and their intake.

Best food sources include: shellfish, fish, lean beef and lamb. Other good sources are dairy products, chicken, egg yolks, dried ginger root, wheatgerm, wholegrain products, beans, legumes, nuts and seeds.

The absorption of zinc is inhibited by iron, which is equally important in pregnancy. This is more of a concern when one, or both, of the nutrients are being taken as a supplement. Do not take these supplements together, perhaps one in the morning, the other in the evening. And try not to take your iron supplement when eating zinc-rich food sources.

If these nutrients are sourced from food, however, absorption is not affected. Nature works wisely and the nutrients are broken down by the body at different rates and absorbed independently of each other. Include zinc and iron-rich food sources in your diet every day to avoid the need for these supplements.

Adding yoghurt to plant-based meals maximises zinc absorption by up to 70 per cent. This is a perk for vegetarians as yoghurt is a great accompaniment to lentil or chickpea dishes.

Iron

Iron and folate are probably the two supplements that you will be recommended to take. While you can aim to ensure your diet is rich in these nutrients, particularly iron, this is an individual decision you will need to discuss with your health practitioner. Iron supplements can have the side effect of constipation, a condition that does not need to be aggravated during pregnancy. Adequate intake of iron-rich foods is your best prevention for avoiding the need for supplements and constipation.

Iron is needed to make the red blood cells that carry oxygen to your baby. It is essential to making the baby's blood supply and increasing your own. An expectant mother's blood volume will increase by up to 30 per cent. This extra blood is needed by the uterus, breasts and other organs and to prepare for blood loss during delivery. Iron is also needed for organ growth. It would be true to say that a woman needs more iron when pregnant than at any other time of her life.

Iron deficiency is very common in pregnant women. Symptoms include tiredness, loss of concentration, low resistance to infection and unhealthy skin and hair. It is also a precursor to anaemia, which is a shortage of haemoglobin (oxygen carriers) in the blood. In more extreme conditions, anaemia can continue after pregnancy and re-occur throughout your lifetime. With its major symptom being fatigue—a tired new mum is simply no fun.

A foetus will never go without the nutrients it requires. If there is not a plentiful supply the placenta will draw on the mother's blood supply for its needs. This is to the detriment of the mother's body if she is not adequately nourished.

If iron-rich foods are not a part of your diet already, they should be introduced immediately. They are an important part of preconception, to build iron levels up, and should continue throughout your entire pregnancy, especially during the second and third trimesters when blood volume is peaking and when most cases of anaemia are diagnosed. Iron levels should be tested each trimester.

Iron is best absorbed from animal products. Some plant foods contain iron but it is in a different form and not as well-absorbed. Vegetarians will need to increase their intake.

Best food sources include: lean red meat (lamb is slightly richer than beef), chicken and turkey, fish and shellfish, egg yolks, legumes and beans, nuts and seeds, dried fruit, spirulina (seaweed), cocoa and Milo, wholegrain products, iron-enriched breakfast cereals and green, leafy vegetables.

The absorption of iron is greatly enhanced when combined with foods rich in vitamin C. These foods must be eaten together and in the same meal. This can be as easy as drinking a glass of orange juice with your meal, or serving dark leafy greens with a piece of steak. You can marinate chicken in lemon juice and herbs, or sprinkle toasted sesame seeds over steamed broccoli. Vegetarians should always aim to eat a food rich in vitamin C with their iron source.

Caffeine hinders or decreases iron absorption so avoid consuming chocolate, tea or coffee with your iron-rich meals. And remember, iron and zinc must always be eaten separately as iron inhibits the absorption of zinc.

Calcium 4 servings Daily

Everyone associates calcium with the pregnancy diet and not surprisingly—a woman's calcium requirement *doubles* during pregnancy. It is crucial for growing strong bones, teeth and nails, vital for the functioning of all muscles, including the heartbeat, as well as blood clotting, nerve development, enzyme activity and the production of colostrum in breastfeeding. Calcium also assists in managing hypertension and diabetes.

Calcium is excreted from the body at a much higher rate during pregnancy, especially when eaten with a high-protein meal. Tofu is an exception to this rule. Iron supplements and tannin (found in black tea) can also restrict the absorption of calcium. The good news is that fresh fruit and vegetables increase absorption and can buffer the protein effect.

Calcium must be included in the diet for the full term of pregnancy, with an even greater demand during the third trimester when baby's bones and teeth are hardening. Your baby is greedy when it comes to its nutritional needs, especially calcium. If there is inadequate supply in the mother's diet, the baby will draw upon her bones. This puts the mother at high risk of developing osteoporosis later in life. Osteoporosis is a condition where bones lose calcium, become fragile and easily fractured. It is the major cause of disability and handicap in Australia.

Calcium deficiency not only raises the concern of osteoporosis, but a severe deficiency can also put you at risk of pre-eclampsia, a condition associated with high blood pressure. Pre-eclampsia can be life-threatening to both mother and baby if not treated immediately. Calcium and magnesium reduce the risk of developing this condition.

Experts recommend three to four servings of calcium per day, but the number of servings are dependent on your sources. If they are not rich sources, you may need more. One serve of calcium equals 250 millilitres (8 fluid ounces) milk, 40 grams (1½ ounces) cheese or 200 grams (7 ounces) yoghurt. Dairy products are undoubtedly the best and most easily absorbed source of calcium. Milk, yoghurt and skim milk powder are the richest food sources.

Best food sources include: dairy products; skim milk powder; hard cheese; dark-green, leafy vegetables; canned salmon and sardines (with bones); sesame seeds (try tahini paste and hummus); most soy products (choose calcium fortified tofu and whole soy beans); wholegrain products, and dried figs, almonds and brazil nuts.

Increasing your calcium intake is very easy. Add low-fat cheese to salads and sandwiches, toss toasted nuts or seeds over salads and steamed vegetables, incorporate skim milk powder into baked goods, soups or smoothies, or simply enjoy a glass of milk.

Calcium does not work alone. It must be properly absorbed and retained by the body for its benefits to be fulfilled. Vitamin D, magnesium and weight-bearing exercise all play a major role in this process.

Vitamin D

Vitamin D helps maximise the benefits of calcium. It transports calcium from the blood into the bones. Without sufficient amounts of vitamin D in the diet, calcium is not properly absorbed. Luckily, deficiency is rare as the best source of vitamin D is sunlight. Women who fully cover their face and body with clothing due to religious or cultural reasons need to ensure their vitamin D is sourced from food.

Best food sources include: egg yolks, parmesan cheese, yoghurt and sardines.

We've mentioned that vitamins and minerals are best sourced from natural foods in their natural state. The presence of calcium and vitamin D from one food source ensures the function of calcium is complete. This is hard to replicate in a supplement, in fact vitamin D supplements can be dangerous during pregnancy.

Magnesium

Magnesium is also vital in obtaining the full benefits of calcium. Magnesium helps the body keep the calcium in the bones. Calcium is easily lost from the body and is excreted in our urine every day. And as mentioned, pregnant women naturally excrete more calcium.

Magnesium is also essential for muscle contractions, including the heartbeat and nerve function. Magnesium reduces the risk of high blood pressure and is prescribed to relieve leg cramps (a common and painful complaint of the second and third trimesters). Magnesium and calcium are also both natural sedatives and a useful remedy if feeling stressed, anxious or irritable.

Best food sources include: milk and skim milk powder; dark, leafy greens, including spinach, rocket, parsley and cabbage; pumpkin seeds, sunflower seeds and fennel seeds; brazil nuts, almonds and walnuts; wholegrain products, including wheatgerm, buckwheat and wholemeal flour and rye bread; bananas; parmesan cheese, and peas.

B-group vitamins

B-group vitamins are another must in the pregnancy diet. They are vital to foetal growth and development; needed for healthy skin, hair, eyes and blood; essential for the nervous system; necessary to break down foods, which releases energy to the body; and are significant in relieving the discomforts of pregnancy such as nausea, fatigue, anaemia, constipation, insomnia and anxiety.

The B-group vitamins are the key players in converting food to fuel. This fuel is used to carry out the body's daily functions. A deficiency in any of the B vitamins can trigger tiredness and fatigue, while severe deficiencies may impair proper foetal development.

Vitamin B12 is especially important. B12 is needed for the production of haemoglobin and DNA (genetic material) and is vital to the development of baby's brain and nervous system. More often than not, anaemia is a result of a deficiency in B12 rather than iron as the two are equally important for healthy blood. B12 is primarily found in animal foods. Vegetarians can rely on dairy products for adequate intake, but vegans need to take extra care and may consider taking a supplement.

Best food sources include: red meat, chicken and turkey, eggs, seafood and low-fat dairy products. Other good sources are wholegrain products, especially wheatgerm; mushrooms; fruits and vegetables; soy products and nuts and seeds.

Vitamin C   1 to 2 servings daily

Vitamin C is required throughout your entire pregnancy and while you don't necessarily need to increase your intake (if adequate), you do need to eat *at least* one rich source per day. The body cannot store vitamin C, nor can your baby, so daily intake is important.

Vitamin C performs many functions during pregnancy. It fights infection by supporting the immune systems of both mother and baby, repairs tissues and heals wounds (for mother after delivery), required for the functioning of all organs, maximises the absorption of iron into the body, is essential for the formation of collagen, promoting skin elasticity (preventing stretch marks), and tones the uterus, enabling it to repair itself more quickly after birth. It also guards against cell mutation, is needed for a healthy placenta, and helps develop strong bones and teeth.

Vitamin C is a water-soluble nutrient so it is easily depleted from foods when exposed to heat and light and is steadily lost in storage. Foods rich in vitamin C are best eaten fresh, uncooked and shortly after purchase. Store these foods in dark, cool places, ideally your fridge.

Vitamin C is found in most red, green and yellow vegetables. Richly-coloured foods indicate higher nutritional value. Deep red tomatoes are bursting with vitamin C while red capsicum has more than three times the amount of vitamin C than its green cousin.

Best food sources include: guava, blackcurrants, red capsicum, dried currants, kiwi fruit, berries (particularly strawberries), papaya, citrus fruits, red cabbage, watercress, Brussels sprouts, broccoli and cauliflower and tomatoes. Breast milk is extremely high in vitamin C so it will be the best source of the nutrient for your baby.

Vitamin C should only be sourced from food sources during pregnancy. Supplements are not recommended as they are thought to be quite dangerous if taken during pregnancy. The body will only break down what it needs from the food source and excrete what it does not need.

omega 3

We have already discussed the importance of essential fatty acids in the pregnancy diet— they play a vital role in every single cell, tissue and organ of the body. Omega 3 is the king of these fatty acids. It keeps the heart in good health. It is needed to produce reproductive hormones, for growth of the placenta and for the formation of collagen for healthy skin. It is a key nutrient in your before, during and after pregnancy diet.

Omega 3 is one of the best foods for your baby's brain. Intake should be increased during the third trimester, when the most rapid growth of the baby's brain occurs. As the brain is not fully developed at birth, it is essential for omega 3 to be continued in the diets of lactating mothers and young infants. Omega 3 is also good for baby's eyes and supports the immune system of the expectant mother. A deficiency may result in under-developed nervous and immune systems in the newborn, making it more susceptible to infections and disease in its infant and adult life.

As with folate and vitamin C, the body cannot produce omega 3. It relies completely on your dietary intake. Fish and seafood are your best sources. Oily fish are the richest choices, with smaller amounts found in white fish.

Best seafood sources include: salmon (fresh, canned and smoked), sardines, good quality canned tuna (not fresh), and calamari.

Flaxseed oil is nature's most potent source of omega 3 and an excellent plant source. One tablespoon per day is just what the doctor ordered. Drizzle over breakfast cereal (before milk is added), steamed vegetables or in salad dressings. It is important to store flaxseed oil in the refrigerator and never cook or directly heat flaxseed oil as nutrients may be damaged. Other plant sources include walnuts, canola and sunflower oil. Generally plant sources are not as easily absorbed or concentrated as animal sources, but they are still beneficial to your diet.

Iodine

Iodine is a nutrient that is beginning to receive more attention regarding its importance in the pregnancy diet. Iodine produces a hormone that regulates mental and physical growth and development. A deficiency can affect normal brain development. Recent studies have shown that an iodine deficiency can affect the development of a baby's brain by up to five to ten IQ points! For adults, iodine prevents goitre and promotes normal functioning of the brain and thyroid gland.

Iodine deficiencies are quite common in Australia, due to a lack of the mineral in this country's soil. Normally rich plant sources (such as barley, bananas and raisins) are not as beneficial as they might once have been, or are, in other countries. For this reason, iodine is best sourced from animal products, with seafood being the richest choice—yet another reason why seafood is so important to the pregnancy diet.

Best food sources include: seafood, eggs and iodised salt. Vegans may need a supplement. Seek advice from your health practitioner if in doubt.

Supplements

Prenatal folic acid, iron, vitamin B12 and calcium are the most commonly prescribed supplements due to their vital roles in reproduction. But, it is a fact that vitamins and minerals are best absorbed and digested by the body from natural food sources. This ensures the right balance of nutrients is obtained but, more importantly, it allows the nutrients to work together, just as nature intended. Nutrients cannot work effectively alone. They work in specific combinations to carry out their functions.

Dietary supplements rarely provide the correct balance or combination. This can cause an imbalance of nutrients in the body that can actually promote a deficiency in another nutrient. If you do add supplements to your diet, ensure it is under the supervision and prescription of a respected health practitioner. There are supplements that must be avoided during pregnancy and these include:

- vitamin A— linked to birth defects in the baby's bones and central nervous system. Vitamin A from food sources is safe as the body will only absorb what it needs
- vitamin C—mega-doses put stress on the kidneys, which are already working overtime during pregnancy
- calcium—can interfere with zinc absorption and unbalance magnesium levels
- iron—a common side effect is constipation.

Dietary supplements overall can be hard to tolerate during the first trimester and can trigger nausea.

Herbs and Spices

Fresh herbs are often underestimated and worth more than a casual appearance as a garnish. Herbs can flavour foods and totally transform a meal. They have substantial nutritional value and many health benefits. They assist with digestive problems, lower cholesterol, stimulate appetite, help prevent disease, nourish the liver and have antiseptic and anti-inflammatory properties and are rich in antioxidants.

Herbs are a healthy substitute for salt, processed sauces or saturated fats used to flavour foods. They marry well with meats in marinades (rosemary and lamb), bring the best out in fruits and vegetables (tomato and basil), are a fabulous finale to stir-fries and salads and are essential for pesto, tabouli and salsas. In fact, herbs are the most simple and tasty way of adding flavour and nutrition to any meal. Seafood particularly benefits from being cooked with herbs. The herbs act as an anti-oxidant and help to preserve essential fatty acids. Adding garlic to seafood can lower blood cholesterol.

A home herb garden is a great way to use more herbs. They are fresh, readily available and totally organic! Parsley, mint and rosemary are the easiest herbs to grow and they are absolutely brimming with nourishment. Try to eat at least one of these varieties every day. Parsley and mint can be added to fresh juices, salads and soups, with mint particularly delicious in desserts or with yoghurt as a savoury side dish. Rosemary, basil and thyme are just as nutritious and versatile and look great in the garden or in pots on a windowsill. See the following table for great uses and benefits of herbs and spices.

VARIETY	GOOD FOR	USED IN
BASIL	nausea, stomach cramps, anxiety, toning heart muscles	best eaten fresh in salads, pesto, pasta, curries, soups, bruschetta and Asian dishes; fabulous with lamb, parmesan cheese, tomatoes and extra-virgin olive oil
CINNAMON	nausea, loss of appetite, digestion, heartburn, circulation, diarrhoea, flatulence, colds and flu, antibacterial properties. Recent studies claim it may help to lower blood sugar levels	desserts, stews, warm milk and baking as a dried and ground spice
CORIANDER	digestion, good source of vitamin A and B-group vitamins, including folate	Asian dishes, salads, noodles, rice and couscous dishes as a fresh herb; goes well with fish, beef, chicken, pork, yoghurt, ginger, garlic and avocado
CUMIN	heartburn, flatulence, lactation. Has sedative properties	Moroccan-inspired dishes; use seed or ground spice
DILL	calms digestion, has soothing qualities	best fresh with fish, poultry or egg dishes and in salads with beetroot, beans, cucumber and potatoes
FENNEL	nausea, bloating, digestion, poor appetite	seeds used in tea infusions, cakes, biscuits, baked potatoes; fresh fennel great with fish
GARLIC	controlling blood pressure, lowering cholesterol, maintaining healthy gut, as remedy for colds and flu	most savoury dishes, good with fish, chicken, lamb, lemon, spinach, basil and parsley
GINGER	nausea, stimulating appetite, blood circulation, hypertension	Asian dishes, vegetable and fruit juices, tea infusions, broths, marinades; ground spice used in baking, middle eastern and Spanish dishes

VARIETY	GOOD FOR	USED IN
MINT	digestion, nausea, vomiting, circulation, heart palpitations. Can relieve stomach cramps and induce sleep	stir-fries, Indian dishes, salads, salsas, marinades, tea infusions; goes with lamb, tomatoes, chickpeas and yoghurt
NUTMEG	nausea	fresh nutmeg grated over cooked spinach, baked pumpkin, rice puddings or desserts made with ginger and honey
OREGANO	ear, nose, throat and lung infections, stimulates digestion	Italian dishes, complements fish, lamb, chicken and tomatoes; use fresh or dried
PARSLEY	anaemia, digestion, fluid retention, constipation, poor appetite, cleansing lungs, liver function, boosting immune system, useful source of iron and vitamin A	tabbouli, salads, soups, casseroles, juices, goes well with fish, beans, eggs, garlic, lemons, lentils, pasta; best eaten fresh
ROSEMARY	heart, blood clotting, digestion, relieving indigestion and wind, rich source of antioxidants	great with lamb, chicken, pork, bread and potatoes; use fresh rosemary when chargrilling meats to counteract cancer-causing substances

Herbs need to be handled with care. They are delicate, bruise easily and, like vegetables, are susceptible to nutritional loss during cooking and storage. If you are purchasing your herbs, wrap them in a paper towel, place in a plastic bag and then store in the fridge. Most herbs will keep for four to five days if stored correctly. Add fresh herbs just prior to serving to minimise nutritional loss.

Spices are just as beneficial in cooking, with infinite varieties, unlimited uses and many therapeutic benefits. Store spices in an airtight container in a dark, cool place. See the table for great herb and spice uses and remedies.

✿ Pregnancy Superfoods

ALMONDS	Rich in protein, zinc, calcium, magnesium, potassium, phosphorus, vitamin E and antioxidants. Good for the brain, heart, nervous system, digestion and blood pressure.
ASIAN GREENS	Great source of folate, antioxidant-rich, no fat, high in fibre plus calcium, beta carotene, potassium and vitamin C.
APRICOTS	Fresh or dried, a high source of dietary fibre and are low GI. Relieves constipation and balances nervous system. Contains vitamins A, B and C, iron, potassium and magnesium.
AVOCADO	Rich in omega 3 and essential amino acids; also contains vitamins B6, C, K and folate. Use as a spread instead of butter.
BANANA	Convenient snack rich in iodine, iron, zinc, potassium, folate and vitamins A, B and E. Known to treat diarrhoea.
BLUEBERRIES	One of the best antioxidant food sources you can eat; very rich in vitamin C, with half a punnet supplying the recommended daily requirement. Good source of fibre, vitamins B6 and E, potassium and bioflavonoids that assist absorption of other fruits. Great for eyesight, healthy kidneys, strong blood capillaries and diarrhoea. Eat half a cup every day!
BRAZIL NUTS	Excellent source of selenium for fertility. Also contain protein, fibre, essential fatty acids, calcium, zinc and B vitamins.
CARROTS	Rich in beta-carotene for eyesight, they treat heartburn, constipation and flatulence and are good for circulation, immunity, skin, hair and nails. One of the few vegetables that is more nutritious when cooked. Raw carrots inhibit activity of listeria by reducing the risk of food poisoning.
CHEESE (hard block varieties, especially parmesan and tasty)	Excellent source of protein, calcium, magnesium, zinc and vitamins D and A. High in saturated fat, so eat in moderation.
CHICKPEAS AND LENTILS	The wonder food! Highly nutritious, great for digestion, hypertension and diabetes. Low in fat, high in protein and fibre, a low GI carbohydrate that contains iron, calcium, magnesium, zinc, B vitamins and essential fatty acids.

DAIRY PRODUCTS— LOW FAT (milk and yoghurt best sources)	Most absorbable source of calcium and contains all essential amino acids. Great source of protein and vitamin B12. Milk is close to being a complete food. Yoghurt aids digestion. Both are rich in magnesium, phosphorus, potassium and vitamins A, B-group and D. Hard cheeses are recommended during pregnancy. Soft cheeses (cottage, cream cheese) have less calcium.
DARK GREEN VEGETABLES (broccoli, spinach, rocket)	Excellent source of folate, calcium and vitamin C. Low-fat, fibre rich, useful sources of beta-carotene, iron, magnesium, potassium. Use minimal water when cooking to retain nutritional value.
DRIED FRUIT	Contain vitamins A, B3 and C, calcium, iron, phosphorus and potassium. Great high-fibre snack, especially prunes, dried apricots and pears.
EGGS	Nature's own vitamin capsule—close to being a complete food. Higher in protein than chicken. Great source of iodine, omega 3, zinc and vitamin D, as well as folate, iron, calcium, selenium, phosphorus, potassium and vitamin A.
FENNEL	Well-known for its healing powers. Aids nausea, vomiting, bloating, stomach cramps and digestion and prevents flatulence. Seeds are the richest source of the plant.
FLAXSEED OIL	Extremely rich in omega 3 and other essential fatty acids. Contains protein, fibre, calcium, vitamins B1, B3 and B6, magnesium, selenium and potassium. Aids constipation. Do not cook flaxseed oil as it can turn rancid. Use in salad dressings, over steamed vegetables, or sprinkle flaxseeds on yoghurt or cereal. Must be stored in refrigerator.
GARLIC	Antibacterial and healing properties. Strengthens immune system, good for blood circulation, colds and flu and general good health.
GINGER	Remedy for nausea and digestion. Boosts circulation and metabolism and provides energy boost. Contains calcium, vitamin B5, magnesium, zinc and potassium.
HERBS (fresh)	Nutritionally packed with protein, fibre, antioxidants, folate, iron, beta carotene, calcium, vitamins A, B2, C and K, magnesium, phosphorus and potassium. The healthiest way to flavour foods, especially parsley, basil, mint and rosemary.

LEAN MEAT (beef, lamb and chicken)	Most absorbable source of iron, containing all essential amino acids. Great source of protein, zinc and vitamin B12.
OATS	The wonder grain. Highly nutritious, a great alternative to wheat and a wise breakfast option. Low GI complex carbohydrate, high in fibre, protein and essential fatty acids. Good source of calcium, magnesium, potassium and folate. Vital to a healthy nervous system and useful for treating diabetes and mild depression.
PEAR	A fabulous food for pregnancy. Calms the digestive system, cleanses, heals and is a good aid for constipation. Low GI.
SEAFOOD (salmon, mussels canned sardines and tuna)	Very important food source during pregnancy. Has the lowest level of saturated fat of all animal proteins. Excellent source of zinc, iodine, omega 3 and vitamin B12. Also contains iron, calcium, B-group vitamins, potassium and phosphorus. Shellfish is the best food source of zinc.
SESAME SEEDS	Very rich source of calcium, protein, vitamin E and fibre. Good for the liver, kidneys, circulation and fatigue.
SUNFLOWER SEEDS	Rich in omega 3 and dietary fibre, with traces of folate, iron, zinc, calcium, magnesium and selenium.
TOFU	The only non-animal source of complete protein. Low in saturated fat and free of cholesterol. Great source of iron, calcium, magnesium phosphorus, potassium, B-group vitamins and dietary fibre. Tofu and tofu products should be eaten in moderation (2–3 servings a week are advised).
WHEATGERM	Fantastic source of zinc. Contains protein, fibre, folate, vitamin B6, potassium and magnesium as well as iron, calcium and essential fatty acids. Have a tablespoon in smoothies or on cereal for breakfast every day.
WHOLEGRAINS	One of the best sources of B-group vitamins and folate. Low GI carbohydrate, useful source of protein and dietary fibre. Also contains calcium, magnesium, zinc, selenium and potassium.

✿ Preconception

If you have made the decision to have a baby, you now have a wonderful opportunity to prime your body for the best possible experience. Beginning pregnancy in excellent health will help to avoid complications, minimise discomforts and eliminate the likelihood of developing any nutritional deficiencies. A well-nourished body really is the foundation for a happy pregnancy.

Preconception is a great opportunity to assess your diet. It is a time to undo any unhealthy eating habits that may have developed. Perhaps you skip breakfast, regularly feast on highly processed foods, or can't live without that caffeine fix. Well, it might be time to make a few minor adjustments. It makes sense to deal with any nutritional deficiencies in preconception rather than when your body is under the demands of a pregnancy. It is important to note that deficiencies in folate and iodine (vital prenatal nutrients) can actually take up to five months to replenish.

You may find it difficult to conceive if you are underweight, under-nourished, or even healthy but with low levels of zinc and protein. Zinc is imperative to fertility in both men and women. And protein is necessary for the development of egg cells in the ovaries and a healthy womb for implantation. Men also need to be in good health as nutritional deficiencies can influence sperm production. A diet rich in vitamins A, B, C, E, selenium and zinc is fundamental to fertility.

It is advised to start a preconception diet up to four months prior to conceiving. This should consist of low GI complex carbohydrates, first-class protein, fresh vegetables and fruit, small amounts of healthy fats and very limited amounts of sugar. There are also a few nutrients that need to be focused on:

1. Folate is crucial in the first six weeks of pregnancy to prevent spina bifida. It can take a couple of months to get folate levels up to the required levels, so the earlier you start eating those green leafy vegetables, the better. A daily intake of 800 milligrams of folate per day is recommended during preconception and the first trimester. If you are unsure of your intake, or fell pregnant without pre-planning, it is advisable to consult your health practitioner and discuss the need for a supplement.

2. Iron is essential throughout your entire pregnancy. If you start your pregnancy with healthy levels and constantly replenish your diet with iron-rich foods, you will avoid the risk of developing anaemia or the need for supplements.

3. Zinc deficiencies can be common, especially for those who don't eat red meat. Zinc is imperative for fertility and often the cause of an inability to conceive.

4.　Calcium　is stored in the bones and these stores can be severely compromised during pregnancy. Ensure your calcium levels are high from the very beginning and maintain them by eating daily three to four servings of calcium-rich foods.

5.　Magnesium　is needed in order to get the full benefits of calcium and protein. It is important in preconception as it retains calcium in the bones, building up your stores for pregnancy.

6.　Vitamin C　boosts and maintains the immune system. It is needed for healthy skin and gums and is involved in the production of hormones.

7.　Essential fatty acids　(especially omega 3) play a key role in fertility and hormone production and are therefore imperative to preconception. Aim to eat at least one of the following every day: oily fish (salmon), avocado, nuts and healthy oils such as flaxseed, grape seed and olive oil.

8.　Iodine　is necessary throughout your entire pregnancy. It is vital for the baby's normal brain development, eyesight and hearing. Iodine deficiencies can be common in countries such as Australia as the soils are low in this essential mineral. Iodine has few rich sources, with the highest from animal products. Vegetarians need to take note of this.

9.　Phosphorus　is needed to manufacture genetic material and so it is very important during the first trimester. Being aware of your intake during preconception will ensure adequate levels. Best food sources include chicken, lamb, salmon, beef, skim milk powder, parmesan cheese, pumpkin seeds and brazil nuts—all good foods for pregnancy.

10.　Selenium　assists fertility through its role in hormone function and sexual development. Rich food sources include brazil nuts, wheatgerm, seafood, chicken, wholemeal and rye bread.

11.　B-group vitamins　are essential so begin your pregnancy with healthy levels.

The recipes in part two are not just for pregnancy. Some, in fact, are great during the preconception period. Among them are the following recipes that will assist your health at this time.

❀ recipes for preconception

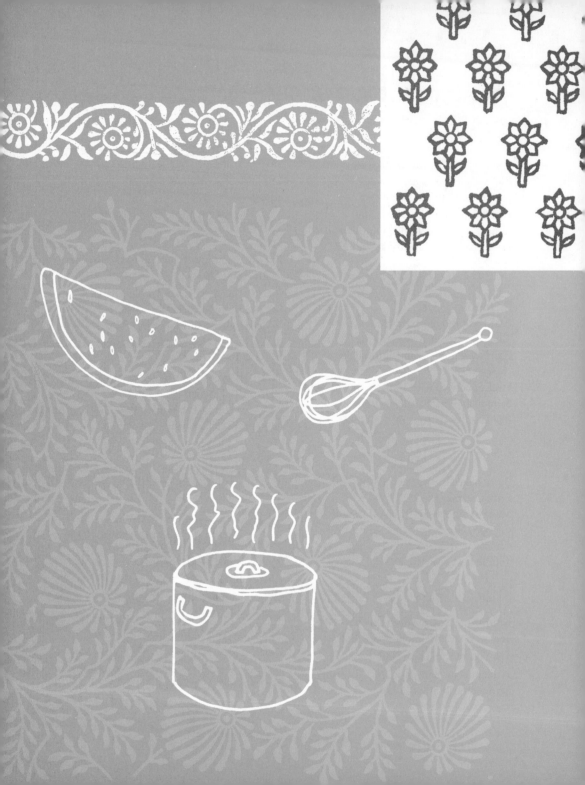

Part Two

Recipes for Pregnancy

✾ About the recipes

Now it's time to head to the kitchen! I have specifically formulated the recipes in this book to assist you through a comfortable pregnancy and to help your baby grow healthily. Each trimester of pregnancy has its own characteristic nutritional requirements and health concerns. The following chapters address these trimester by trimester and provide food advice and remedies. Each recipe also states what you and your baby can gain from the ingredients to meet both of your needs at this particular stage of foetal development.

While the recipes have been devised according to the requirements of a given trimester, they are all essentially nutrient rich. So if you have a favourite, by all means eat it throughout your pregnancy. My recipes for drinks, snacks, ways with bread and side dishes towards the end of this part of the book should be enjoyed for the full term.

Within the trimesters, recipes are divided into the following sections: breakfast, light meals, mains and sweet things. As you know, breakfast is the most important meal of the day, but during pregnancy this is even more so. You and your baby require a constant supply of energy and when you wake in the morning you need to refuel your body.

The light meal recipes are perfect for both lunch and dinner options, particularly towards the end of your term, when you'll probably prefer more frequent, smaller meals. Light meals includes soups, which are a fabulous creation as nutrients normally lost during cooking are retained in the broth. You can also make large quantities of soup and freeze individual portions for those days when you are too tired or busy to cook.

A few recipe notes

Temperatures can differ from oven to oven. When I was testing these recipes I used a gas cook top and an electric oven set on fan-forced. I prefer fan-forced as it takes less time to heat up and the food seems to cook more quickly and evenly, especially cakes and muffins. If I noticed that the was food browning too quickly or too much, I simply switched back to a conventional setting. If you only have a conventional oven, you may need to increase the temperature by 10°C/25°F and add another 10 to 15 minutes to the cooking time.

Most of the recipes serve two adults, unless otherwise specified. It is very easy to increase or decrease portion sizes by halving or doubling the ingredients as required. All the recipes were made with low-fat dairy products. The olive oil used was extra virgin. The soy sauce was always salt-reduced and I use only wholemeal flour in my food.

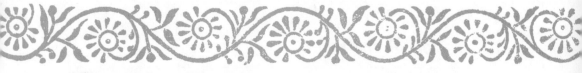

❋ first trimester weeks 0 to 13

The first trimester is the one most influenced by diet. The foetus is at its most vulnerable and is affected by everything that it is exposed to during the first six weeks of pregnancy. In addition, the most important phases in the development of all major organs and external structures take place during this period. Make every mouthful nutritionally rich and aim to avoid junk food, processed food and anything that contains additives and preservatives.

Protein is very important, as are complex carbohydrates. Both nutrients provide energy. Foods high in dietary fibre should be eaten daily to prevent constipation, and get into the habit of eating loads of fresh vegetables and fruit.

The essential nutrients needed at this time are: folate, iron, zinc, b-group vitamins (with focus on vitamin B12), calcium and magnesium, vitamin C, phosphorus and vitamin A (from food sources only).

PROGRESSION OF BABY

WHAT'S HAPPENING	WHAT'S NEEDED
Embryo resembles human form and becomes a foetus	
Neural tube develops and closes down six weeks after last menstruation	folate, B12, B6, phosphorus
All major organs developed and ready to mature	zinc, calcium, protein
Central nervous system develops	b-group (especially B6 and B12)
Blood cells multiply	iron, folate, vitamins B5 and B12
Heart starts beating. Blood circulation begins	calcium, protein, iron, zinc
Brain and muscle coordination	calcium, vitamin B5, potassium, sodium
External structures form. Bones start to harden	calcium, magnesium, zinc, protein, vitamin C
Limbs grow rapidly. Muscles begin to develop	calcium, protein, carbohydrates
Skin, hair and ears form	selenium, vitamins B2, B3, D and A
Eyes develop in the first eight weeks	vitamins D, A and B2 for great vision

Progression of mother

WHAT'S HAPPENING	WHAT'S NEEDED
Body prepares for pregnancy, internally but not noticeably	
Pregnancy hormones produced. Increased progesterone can trigger fatigue, constipation and digestive problems	vitamins A, D, E and K, zinc, omega 3, selenium, fibre. Eat small, regular meals
Placenta growing	complete balance of all nutrients
Blood volume increasing	protein, iron, folate, vitamin B12

Common complaints of the first trimester

Fatigue/tiredness

Tiredness, fatigue and nausea are the main symptoms of the first trimester. Your body is adjusting to its new status and working overtime to sustain the pregnancy, support your growing baby and maintain your own good health. It is no wonder you feel tired!

Fatigue is aggravated by nutrient deficiencies and can indicate inadequate protein or iron in the diet. As with most symptoms, a complete and balanced diet with lots of rest is the most effective remedy. Listen to your body; if you are tired, stop and rest.

Energy levels should return by the end of the first trimester, although tiredness may return in the third. Eat small, regular wholesome meals to maintain blood sugar levels and drink plenty of fluids. To fight fatigue:

- eat foods rich in protein and iron
- include low GI complex carbohydrates to promote a gradual release of energy
- eat regularly (every two to three hours) to boost energy and control blood sugar levels
- drink lots of water
- avoid sugar and caffeine
- eat lots of fresh, raw vegetables and vegetable juices
- eat fruit in moderation to control blood sugar levels.

Nausea/morning sickness

Morning sickness (or nausea) is the most talked about symptom of the first trimester. It usually subsides by the second trimester, but for a few unfortunate mums-to-be, it can continue for the entire pregnancy. Despite its name, morning sickness can occur at any time of the day.

Surprisingly, food will help to overcome and relieve nausea. It is not certain what causes nausea during pregnancy, although low blood sugar levels can certainly trigger it. Preventing nausea is without a doubt the best way of dealing with it. You can do this by eating small, regular meals or grazing on nutritious snacks to maintain blood sugar levels.

Obstetricians claim that well-nourished women are generally less inclined to suffer from nausea, particularly those with a diet rich in the B-group vitamins. Vitamins B2, B6 and B12 are very good for treating nausea and preventing the condition all together. Foods rich in these vitamins include bread, rice, cereals, legumes, nuts, yeast, Vegemite and Marmite, eggs, lean meat, chicken, fish, green leafy vegetables, milk and yoghurt.

Tips to overcoming nausea include:

- eating small, regular meals
- avoiding fried, fatty, spicy or sugary foods—in this instance 'spicy' means chilli or dramatic heat-inducing spices, spices such as cumin, fennel, ginger, coriander and turmeric are invaluable when it comes to dealing with nausea and digestive problems
- Increasing complex carbohydrates and combining with high-protein foods, i.e. spaghetti bolognaise, Vegemite/Marmite on toast or toast spread with hummus, chicken noodle soup
- having a high protein/carbohydrate snack just before sleeping, e.g. glass of milk and a cookie
- eating a dry cracker or cookie upon waking and before rising—don't rush out of bed
- drinking lots of fluid, especially fresh fruit and vegetable juices and water—fresh juices are a great way of ensuring vitamin and mineral intake if solids are proving a problem
- Eating and drinking separately. Try not to drink with meals or solid food.

47

foods to ease nausea

Starchy carbohydrates	Plain boiled rice, pasta, potatoes and bread
Ginger	Fresh ginger root is more effective than the ground spice. Use in fresh fruit and vegetable juices, teas, stir fries and baking
Cinnamon	Relieves diarrhoea, nausea and loss of appetite. Mix into warm milk before sleeping
Fennel	Seeds are most effective. Infuse in boiling water for a remedial tea; chew raw seeds or use in baking, soups and stews
Fresh basil	Add fresh to salads, soups and pasta
Fresh mint	Effective remedy for vomiting. Use in salads, salsas and fresh juice
Lemon and lime	Their sharp flavours can excite a bland and changing palate. Try a good squeeze of fresh lemon or lime juice in a glass of carbonated water
Sour fruits	Green apples, grapefruit and green grapes. Many women claim sour-tasting fruits relieve symptoms
Carrots, oranges and Raspberries	Freshly juiced allows easier absorption by the body. Drink carrot and fresh ginger juice daily to ward off nausea

Remedies for nausea seem to be very individual. What works for others may not work for you. Many claim ginger has no effect; others swear by it. Fennel seeds are highly praised.

Protein can be hard to tolerate when nauseous but due to its importance in the pregnancy diet, intake must be maintained. If the smell and taste of high-protein foods such as meat or fish is off-putting, try disguising it with other flavours to overcome the aversion or ask someone else to prepare the meal for you. Garlic, ginger, fennel and lime are terrific at disguising flavours!

In more severe cases, some women find it hard to eat anything at all. It is important to try to eat small portions to keep your energy levels up and to provide fuel for your growing baby. Vegemite or Marmite on wholegrain toast seems to be a winner and is often the only food that nauseous women can tolerate. This could be attributed to the high content of b-group vitamins in both the spread and the bread. It also provides reasonable amounts of calcium and protein.

Pasta is another popular option. Serve with a light, tomato-based sauce or even your favourite bolognaise topping. Try adding a teaspoon of ground cinnamon to bolognaise sauce—the flavour is amazing and cinnamon can relieve nausea. Plain basmati or brown rice cooked in protein-rich chicken stock is another good choice.

If none of the above, healthier options appeal, try nibbling on dry salted crackers. Many women claim that foods high in salt are helpful. If this is the case for you, be sure to drink plenty of water throughout the day to help control sodium levels. Too much salt in the diet can promote fluid retention and high blood pressure and affect kidney function.

Loss of nutrients is a concern in the more severe cases of morning sickness, with vomiting and diarrhoea flushing food and its goodness from the body. Iron is a particular concern as it is absorbed in the stomach. Contact your health practitioner if these symptoms persist. Taking dietary supplements may be necessary if you cannot keep any food down.

Dehydration is another concern when vomiting. As hard as it may be, you must try to keep up your fluid intake. Take small, regular sips of water and, if you can stomach food, consume those with high water content. The best sources are fruits and vegetables such as melons, lettuce and citrus fruits.

If solid foods are proving too much then opt for fresh juices, healthy smoothies and nourishing broths. They are easy to digest and a great source of nutrition. Chicken soup is an old favourite and very high in protein.

food aversions

You may start to experience aversions to foods that have never affected you before your pregnancy. The smell, taste and even the sight of specific foods can bring on nausea. This is due to those hormones again. You may also notice a shift in your senses, either heightened or dulled, as well as a change in your palate. Some women can only withstand bland foods; others find that all foods taste bland and need more challenging, zingy flavours.

Many women claim that protein is particularly hard to stomach during the first few months of pregnancy. Protein is an essential nutrient so you need to try and find a way to consume your daily intake. Try to disguise protein sources with other flavours: add cheese to omelettes, braise beef with spices and starchy vegetables, or reap the rewards of seafood without the fishy flavour in a creamy leek and herb fish pie.

If fruit and vegetables become unappealing, try juicing them. They may become more palatable and easier to take in liquid form.

food cravings

These tend to be experienced in the first four months of pregnancy and are more often than not an indication of your body's nutritional needs. It could be assumed that food cravings are experienced during the first trimester as the body takes check on what nutrients it might be lacking in or needs to stock up on so it can maintain a healthy pregnancy for the full term. With this in mind, you may be surprised to hear that most cravings are healthy cravings.

Many women crave fresh orange juice or foods rich in vitamin C. Others seek dairy products, indicating a need for calcium. You may crave complex carbohydrates as your body asks for more fuel and energy. Listen to your body: rest when you are tired, exercise when you are energised and eat when you are hungry.

If your cravings are for unhealthy foods such as sugar, this can be an indication of a need for more complex carbohydrates. Aim to opt for healthy options to satisfy these cravings, such as a wholesome muffin, dried fruit or a fresh fruit smoothie, which can be a healthy alternative to ice-cream. Most food aversions and cravings subside after the first trimester.

fainting, dizziness and headaches

Low blood pressure or low blood sugar levels can trigger headaches or dizziness. Fainting is not as common as dizziness but is caused by the same symptoms. All three conditions may be experienced throughout your entire pregnancy, but can usually be controlled by following these general guidelines for a healthy pregnancy diet.

- Eat small, regular meals and healthy snacks—almonds are particularly good. Try to eat every two to three hours.
- Maintain your iron intake and vitamin E, which can help circulation.
- Vitamin C is known to relieve headaches. Eat an orange or a vitamin C-rich fruit salad.
- Drink plenty of fluids.

Dental problems

Believe it or not, bleeding gums are a symptom of pregnancy. They are triggered by hormones and increased blood volume which softens the gums, making them more susceptible to bleeding and infection. New studies are indicating that gum disease may cause premature births. Gum disease increases the production of chemicals and proteins that are said to induce labour.

Dental problems can begin in the first trimester and continue for the full term of pregnancy. It is therefore important to maintain healthy teeth and gums throughout. Strict oral hygiene is an absolute must, together with a diet rich in calcium, protein and vitamins B, C and D. Low levels of any of these nutrients can exacerbate the problem. Gum disease can be due to a vitamin C deficiency, while increased calcium intake can prevent bleeding.

Sugar intake and sugary foods should be limited, if not avoided. Regular meals or snacks with sugar means sugar is constantly present in the mouth.

Foods for healthy teeth include:

- lots of fresh (preferably raw) vegetables, especially dark leafy greens, broccoli and capsicum
- fruits high in vitamin C, including citrus, berries, kiwi fruit, apples
- wholegrains and their products
- all legumes and dried peas
- dairy products
- tinned salmon and sardines
- almonds and sesame seeds.

51

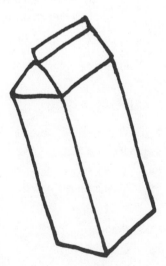

❀ recipes for first trimester
weeks 1 to 13

Best-ever Bircher Muesli

This is a healthy adaptation of the traditional bircher muesli. Its beneficial combination of grains and dairy make it a complete source while the low GI ingredients make this a perfect breakfast to get you through the day.

1 cup rolled oats

1 tbs each of wheatgerm and oat bran

2 tbs chopped nuts (any combination of almonds, hazelnuts, sunflower,

pepitas, sesame seeds)

⅓ cup fresh or frozen blueberries

⅓ cup low-fat berry yoghurt

½ cup (120 ml/4 fl oz) apple juice (freshly juiced or no-added sugar)

low-fat, skim or soy milk

Place dry ingredients in a cereal bowl. Add berries, yoghurt and apple juice, mix well. Pour over enough milk to cover muesli. Seal with cling wrap and refrigerate for at least one hour but best if left overnight to allow the flavours to blend and make the grains easier to digest. Eat as is or add a little more milk or yogurt if desired.

tip *You can prepare bulk quantities of the dry ingredients and store in an airtight container in the pantry. To make, scoop one heaped cup of dry ingredients per person into a bowl and continue as above.*

GOOD SOURCE OF: *calcium, protein, fibre, vitamins C, D, E, B6 and B12, folate, potassium, magnesium, zinc, phosphorus, essential fatty acids, antioxidants*

GOOD FOR MOTHER: *sustained energy, digestion, fatigue, hypertension, constipation, circulation, skin elasticity, healthy heart and blood, nourishing placenta, diabetes*

GOOD FOR BABY: *fuelling foetal growth, development of neural tube, brain, spine and central nervous system, manufacture of genetic material, formation of major organs, external structures, skin, hair and eyes, heartbeat*

Boiled Eggs with Vegemite Soldiers

A simple but effective breakfast to deal with the two most common complaints of the first trimester: fatigue and nausea. How to cook the perfect boiled egg has been under contention for many years and will be for many more. Yet there are two factors agreed on by cooks and chefs alike: always use fresh eggs, and bring them to room temperature before cooking—chilled eggs may crack during cooking.

2 eggs, preferably biodynamic

2 slices wholegrain toast

Vegemite or Marmite

Fill a medium saucepan with enough cold water to completely cover the eggs. Gently place the eggs into the water. Bring water to a simmer or very gentle boil. Cook eggs for 4–8 minutes. Start timing when water begins to simmer.

While the eggs are cooking, toast the wholegrain bread and spread with Vegemite. Now is the time to reminisce a little. Cut your toast into three even pieces, affectionately referred to as soldiers. Remove eggs from pan and briefly plunge eggs into cold water. This will stop the cooking process but will not cool the eggs internally.

Serve eggs in eggcups and dip soliders into the yolk for a double hit of vitamin B! Serves 1.

GOOD SOURCE OF: *vitamins A, D and B12, folate, protein, iron, zinc, iodine, omega 3, calcium, selenium, potassium, fibre*

GOOD FOR MOTHER: *nausea, fatigue, digestion, fertility, healthy blood, anaemia, production of collagen, energy source, boosting immune system*

GOOD FOR BABY: *development of all major organs and circulatory systems, cell growth, eyesight, strong healthy bones and teeth, haemoglobin production*

fruit salad with the works

This breakfast is beneficial during the first and third trimesters, as well as lactation. It is a light, satisfying meal that will keep you energised throughout the entire morning. It may be useful for those who are experiencing nausea or aversions to protein as the nuts and yoghurt are terrific sources. During the third trimester it is not going to overfill you. The combination of ingredients is fantastic for the digestive, immune and nervous systems. It helps prepare your body for birth and the production of colostrum.

>   any combination of apples, bananas, blueberries, raspberries, strawberries,
>   kiwi fruits, mangoes, oranges, pears
>   ½ cup low-fat yoghurt
>   ½ cup natural almonds, roughly chopped
>   1 tbs wheatgerm

Thoroughly wash fruit. Chop into bite-sized pieces and mix in a serving bowl. Top with yoghurt and nuts and sprinkle with wheatgerm. Serves 1.

55

tip *Smaller portions make an excellent snack.*

GOOD SOURCE OF: *vitamins A, C and E, fibre, calcium, magnesium, potassium, phosphorus, folate, zinc, protein, essential fatty acids, antioxidants*

GOOD FOR MOTHER: *constipation, skin elasticity, fluid retention, lactation, food aversions, fatigue, cleansing, growing placenta, immune system, digestion, hypertension, good health*

GOOD FOR BABY: *development of brain, lungs, muscles, healthy hair, skin, fat and central nervous system, cell reproduction, protecting against cell damage, strong bones and teeth*

Stewed Pears and Yoghurt

Pears are the perfect breakfast fruit. They help cleanse and calm the digestion system and yoghurt and spices are effective remedies for nausea. This is a light breakfast that even the most nauseous should be able to tolerate. You can also refrigerate for an easily digestible snack or light dessert.

> **2 ripe pears**
>
> **½ cup (120 ml /4 fl oz) water**
>
> **2 tsp mixed spice**

Chop pears into 2-cm (¾-inch) cubes. Place water and spices into a small saucepan and bring to the boil. Add pears and reduce heat to a simmer. Cover and cook for 5 minutes.

Serve warm with yoghurt or as an accompaniment to cereals for breakfast. Delicious poured over rolled oats and soaked overnight. Serves 1.

GOOD SOURCE OF: *protein, calcium, vitamins B12 and B2, magnesium, potassium, fibre*

GOOD FOR MOTHER: *nausea, digestion, diabetes, healthy bone structure*

GOOD FOR BABY: *development of all major organs, skin, hair, ears and eyes*

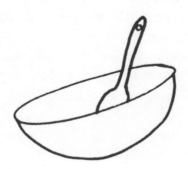

folate-friendly omelette

Eggs are so nourishing and when combined with the goodness of dark, leafy greens and fresh herbs you have an incredibly healthy meal. This omelette contains all the nutrients required for the first vital phases of your baby's development.

> 3 eggs, preferably biodynamic
>
> cracked black pepper
>
> 2 shallots, finely chopped
>
> ½ cup rocket or spinach, roughly chopped
>
> ½ cup fresh parsley, finely chopped
>
> 2 tbs parmesan cheese, grated
>
> 2 tbs chopped chives (optional)

Crack eggs into a bowl, add 1 tablespoon water, season with black pepper and whisk together. Heat a non-stick frying pan over medium–high heat. If your frying pan tends to stick, add 1 tbs of olive oil and swirl to coat. Add egg mixture and tilt the pan to spread evenly over the base. Immediately scatter remaining ingredients over the omelette base. When the omelette edges begin to curl up, use a spatula and gently fold in half and cook for another 2–3 minutes, or until cooked through. Serves 1.

tip *Place omelette on a piece of lavish or mountain bread and roll up for a takeaway wrap. You can even add 2–3 lightly steamed asparagus spears to the wrap for an extra nutrient boost of green.*

GOOD SOURCE OF: *folate, calcium, protein, vitamins A, B12, C, D and K, zinc, iodine, selenium, phosphorus, potassium, omega 3*

GOOD FOR MOTHER: *overall good health, fatigue, building protein, iron and calcium stores, boosting immune system, skin elasticity, fertility*

GOOD FOR BABY: *development of major organs, circulatory and nervous system, formation of external structures, eyes, hair, skin and ears, growth of placenta*

Tuna and Brown Rice Salad

This dish can be pre-made and is the perfect 'portable' lunch. It is packed with
B vitamins, helpful in warding off nausea, as is the protein/carbohydrate combination.
These ingredients also promotes healthy blood and circulation. Brown rice is more
nutritious than white, but it does have a higher GI rating. If you are considered high
risk for gestational diabetes, please substitute brown with basmati or doongara rice.

½ cup brown rice

½ avocado

1 x 185 g (6 oz) can tuna in springwater

2 shallots, finely sliced

½ cup diced beetroot, cooked

½ cup thinly sliced fennel

1 tomato diced (or roasted tomato for more intense flavour)

½ cup chopped fresh parsley

cracked black pepper

1 tbs flaxseed oil

Cook rice according to its packet directions. Once cooked, place in a large salad
bowl and while warm, scoop the avocado into the rice and mix through. The heat will
slightly melt the avocado into a creamy consistency.

Add remaining salad ingredients. Season with black pepper and drizzle with the
flaxseed oil. Toss to combine and dress all ingredients.

GOOD SOURCE OF: *vitamins A, C, E, and B-group, folate, omega 3, protein,
potassium, carbohydrates*
GOOD FOR MOTHER: *nausea, circulation, fatigue, constipation, digestion, immunity,
healthy blood*
GOOD FOR BABY: *development of brain and central nervous system, nourishing
major organs including the liver, heart and skin, encouraging foetal growth*

Rainbow Salad

A foolproof way of serving up a nutritionally balanced meal is to include every colour of the rainbow on your plate, hence the name of this salad. It is fantastic for the health of your liver and your blood. This salad is recommended throughout your pregnancy.

1 carrot, grated

½ beetroot, grated

1 zucchini, grated

2 shallots, sliced

1 tomato or ½ red capsicum, diced

½ cup parsley, chopped

½ avocado, sliced

⅓ cup grated tasty cheese

large handful baby rocket or spinach leaves

dressing:

1 tbs grape seed oil

1 tsp lemon juice

cracked black pepper

59

Pour the grape seed oil and lemon juice in a large salad bowl. Whisk together and season with pepper. Prepare all salad ingredients, noting that all are served raw. Add to the bowl and combine.

tip *To add a high-quality protein for a nutritionally balanced meal, toss in any of the following or serve on the side: canned tuna or salmon; chargrilled salmon fillet flaked into bite-sized pieces; cooked chicken breast, shredded; chickpeas, cannellini beans or mixed beans; tofu cubes, lightly grilled.*

GOOD SOURCE OF: *vitamins A, C, E, K and B-group, folate, potassium, calcium, magnesium, fibre*

GOOD FOR MOTHER: *overall good health, anaemia, fatigue, liver function, fluid retention, constipation, leg cramps, hypertension, digestion, increased blood supply, muscle contractions, healthy skin, hair and eyes, immune system, nourishing placenta*

GOOD FOR BABY: *development of major organs, skin, eyes and body fat, brain and muscle coordination, formation and hardening of external structures, production of body cells and DNA*

fennel and rocket salad

Parsley, beans and rocket are all good sources of folate. For maximum absorption, folate must be eaten with vitamin B12. Parmesan cheese does contain this nutrient, but I recommend serving this salad with a vitamin B12-rich lamb, chicken, pork, white fish or egg dish. This salad goes exceptionally well with grilled pork.

100 g (3½ oz) fresh green beans, cut in half

½ cup fennel, finely sliced

½ cup continental parsley, finely chopped

large handful of baby rocket leaves

⅓ cup fresh parmesan cheese, thinly shaved

dressing:

1 tbs flaxseed or extra virgin olive oil

1 tbs balsamic vinegar

cracked black pepper

Steam beans for 1–2 minutes. Remove from steamer and place into a salad bowl. Add all remaining ingredients. Top with thinly grated slices of parmesan cheese.

Whisk together the flaxseed oil and balsamic vinegar and season with black pepper. Dress salad just prior to serving.

GOOD SOURCE OF: *folate, calcium, vitamins A, B and C.*

GOOD FOR MOTHER: *digestion, nausea, fluid retention, strong blood vessels, healthy skin, blood, liver and kidney function, formation of DNA and body cells*

GOOD FOR BABY: *early development of brain, spinal cord and central nervous system, reducing risk of birth defects, muscle contractions*

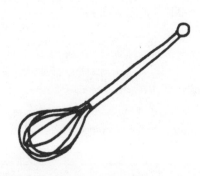

chicken and spring vegetable soup

Chicken soup is always a winner, especially when combined with young, fresh spring vegetables. This soup may assist those experiencing nausea and aversions to protein as the sweet-tasting vegetables do well to disguise the chicken. Finely shred the chicken and you will hardly even notice the taste or texture, and your body will get the nourishment it needs. This recipe also provides a good dose of the ever-important folate, which reduces the risk of birth defects.

2 chicken breasts

6 cups (1½ litres/2 pints 8 fl oz) chicken stock, homemade or low-salt

2 tbs olive oil

1 large leek, sliced

1 zucchini, sliced

zest and juice from 1 lemon

200 g (7 oz) frozen peas, thawed

1 fresh corn cob, kernels removed

1 medium head broccoli

100 g (3½ oz) sugar snap peas or asparagus

1 cup fresh mixed herbs—basil, chives, parsley, mint, thyme, chervil or
    tarragon

61

Poach chicken breasts in 2 cups of chicken stock. Simmer for 5–8 minutes, or until cooked through. Remove from stock and reserve stock for use in the soup.

You will need a large stockpot with a lid. Heat 1 tablespoon of oil over a medium heat. Add leek and cook for 2–3 minutes. Cover and allow to gently simmer for a further 2 minutes. The leek will release a liquid and sweat a little, which will soften and sweeten it. Add zucchini and lemon zest. Stir through and cook for another 2 minutes. Add peas and corn, then stir-fry for a minute or so before adding the stock and lemon juice. Cover with lid and simmer for a couple of minutes.

Shred the chicken breasts, chop broccoli into bite-sized pieces, string the sugar snap peas/trim the asparagus and chop the herbs.

Now add the broccoli and the chicken to the soup. Simmer for 2 minutes before adding the sugar snap peas/asparagus and fresh herbs. Stir through for a final minute to slightly blanch the sugar snap peas/asparagus. You want the green vegetables to retain their nutrients and a nice crunch.

Season generously with cracked black pepper and serve. Serves 4.

GOOD SOURCE OF: *protein, iron, selenium, phosphorus, potassium, zinc, fibre, vitamins A, C, K and B-group, especially folate*

GOOD FOR MOTHER: *nausea, fatigue, food aversions, constipation, digestion, fluid retention, healthy skin, heart and blood, blood sugar levels, growing placenta, fertility, low-fat*

GOOD FOR BABY: *development of neural tube, spine, nervous system and eyes, growth of cells, skin, hair and ears, general foetal growth*

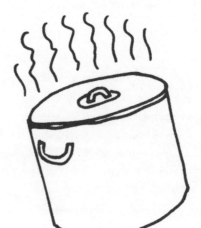

Green Soup

You won't have any problems eating your greens with this recipe. It is brimming with goodness, especially folate, which is crucial during the first trimester. The chicken stock serves as an easily digestible form of protein, useful to those dealing with nausea. Enjoy for lunch or dinner, and serve with wholegrain bread.

2 tbs olive oil

½ bulb fennel, finely sliced (reserving fronds)

1 brown onion, finely chopped

3 cloves garlic

2 sticks celery, diced

1 zucchini, diced

100 g (3½ oz) green beans, diced

1 medium broccoli head, cut into small florets

1 cup frozen peas, thawed

4 cups (1 litre/1 pint 12 fl oz) chicken stock

2 bay leaves

1 sachet bouquet garni

½ bunch silverbeet, roughly chopped (leaves only, white stems removed)

½ cup fresh basil or parsley

freshly grated parmesan cheese

Heat oil in a large saucepan. Add fennel, onion and garlic and cook for 5 minutes, or until onions and fennel have softened. Add remaining vegetables, with the exception of the silverbeet. Add chicken stock, bay leaves, bouquet garni and season with black pepper.

Bring soup to the boil, then reduce heat, cover and simmer for 5 minutes.
Add silverbeet, cover the saucepan and simmer for another 5 minutes.

Spoon into serving bowls and sprinkle with fresh herbs, fennel fronds and parmesan cheese.

This soup can be pureed in a food processor for a thicker texture. Cooked, shredded chicken or cannelini beans can be added for extra protein or a more substantial meal. Add these ingredients to the soup a few minutes before serving. Potatoes can be added if using as a remedy for nausea. Parboil potatoes and add to recipe with vegetables.

GOOD SOURCE OF: *protein, calcium, vitamins C, A, K and B-group including folate, fibre*

GOOD FOR MOTHER: *nausea, fatigue, digestion, food aversions, constipation, healthy blood, immunity*

GOOD FOR BABY: *early development stages of brain, spine and central nervous system, reducing risk of spina bifida, early formation of skin, hair, eyes, muscle contractions*

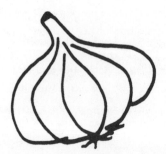

Herbed Chicken Baguette

Protein is essential during pregnancy. Without it, your baby's growth will be greatly compromised. Chicken is a high-quality protein sources and this recipe is a healthy way to flavour and tenderise the meat. I like to cook a batch of the herbed chicken on the weekend for my mid-week lunch fillings. This recipe is also perfect for picnics.

2 chicken breast fillets

1 wholegrain baguette, cut into two
    serving portions

½ avocado

1 tomato, sliced

1 cucumber, thinly sliced diagonally

handful of rocket leaves

marinade:

1 tsp mixed dried herbs

juice of 1 fresh lemon or lime

1 clove garlic, crushed

2 tsp olive oil

Prepare the marinade by combining the herbs, lemon juice, garlic and olive oil.

Trim chicken of all visible fat. Cut the breast horizontally into two thin slices. Do this by placing the knife parallel to the chopping board and slicing through the fillet, cutting along the length of the breast. The result is two thin fillets of roughly the same shape and size. Rinse under cold water and pat dry with a paper towel.

Place the chicken in the prepared marinade, turning a couple of times to coat evenly. Set aside for 20–30 minutes, or longer if possible. A longer marinating time is always beneficial, but in this recipe it is not imperative.

Generously spread the two baguettes with avocado and fill with the tomato, cucumber and rocket leaves. While you grill or barbeque chicken fillets. Place one fillet into each baguette.

65

GOOD SOURCE OF: *protein, omega 3, selenium, vitamin E and B-group including folate, fibre*

GOOD FOR MOTHER: *fatigue, anaemia, digestion, skin elasticity, iron absorption, increased blood supply, healthy skin, hair and eyes, fluid retention, hypertension, fertility, nourishing placenta*

GOOD FOR BABY: *development of brain, muscles, bones, skin, fat, major organs and central nervous system, promoting healthy cells, formation of eyes, strengthening immune system*

Brazil Nut Burgers

These burgers are delicious, versatile and very nourishing. Five of the seven ingredients are pregnancy superfoods. This recipe was devised for the first trimester, but considering its goodness it should be eaten throughout your entire pregnancy.

1 cup cooked chickpeas

2 carrots, grated

⅔ cup brazil nuts

⅓ cup (80 ml/3 fl oz) salt-reduced tamari (wheat-free soy sauce)

1 egg

½ cup (125 ml/4 fl oz) lemon juice

½ cup fresh parsley, chopped

½ cup wheatgerm

Preheat oven to 180°C/350°F. Line a baking tray with baking paper.

Place chickpeas, carrots and nuts in food processor and blend until finely chopped. Add tamari, egg and lemon juice, then process again. Finally, add fresh herbs and wheatgerm and blend to combine. If the mixture is not clinging together, add an extra tablespoon of lemon juice or water.

Mould dessert spoon scoops of the mixture into patties and place on the prepared baking tray. Bake for 20–25 minutes, or until golden brown.

tip *Serve warm with yoghurt and a green salad or cold as an energising snack or as a burger in a wholemeal bread roll with yoghurt, tomato slices and mixed salad leaves. Form into small balls rather than patties when cooking and serve as a healthy pre-dinner snack with yoghurt or sweet chilli sauce.*

GOOD SOURCE OF: *selenium, protein, iron, calcium, magnesium, potassium, vitamins C and B-group, fibre, beta-carotene, essential fatty acids*

GOOD FOR MOTHER: *vegetarians, fertility, fatigue, immunity, skin elasticity, hormone production, constipation, digestion, fatigue, healthy blood and placenta, cell growth*

GOOD FOR BABY: *development of brain, spine, organs and eyes, nervous and immune systems, strong bones, teeth and nails*

Thai-style Steamed Mussels

Mussels are an amazing source of zinc, iodine and selenium. These nutrients are essential for reproduction and cell production and yet they are the nutrients we are most deficient in, mainly because they have limited food sources. Luckily, mussels pack a punch with all three. Mussels only take a few minutes to cook and are hard to spoil. If you are experiencing reflux and heartburn you might want to leave out the chilli.

2 small sweet potatoes, scrubbed clean

700 g (1 lb 8 oz) black mussels

2 tbs fish sauce

1 tbs honey

1 tbs olive oil

½ cup water

3 shallots, finely sliced

3 garlic cloves, finely sliced

½ red chilli, seeds removed and finely diced

1 cup mixed fresh herbs (basil, mint, coriander and chives)

2 tbs lime juice

extra lime wedges to serve

67

Wash and chop the sweet potato into 1-cm (⅖-inch) cubes. Cook in a medium saucepan of boiling water for 10 minutes, or until tender. Drain and set aside.

Place mussels in a colander and rinse under cold, running water. Scrub mussel shells to remove any barnacles and pull out the hairy tufts or 'beards'. Rinse again with cold water and drain.

Combine the fish sauce and honey in a small cup.

Use a large saucepan or wok with a tight-fitting lid. Place oil, water, shallots, garlic and chilli in the pan and bring to the boil. Add the prepared mussels, cover securely with the lid and cook for 1–2 minutes. Shake the pan once or twice. Take off the lid and add the fish sauce and honey. Stir through and discard any mussels that are still securely closed.

Add the sweet potato, herbs and lime juice. Stir thoroughly to mix ingredients and cook for a further minute or two.

Divide mussels into deep serving bowls and pour over the cooking broth.

Serve with steamed rice and a big bowl of steamed green vegetables for extra folate.

GOOD SOURCE OF: *zinc, iodine, omega 3, selenium, protein, calcium, potassium, phosphorus, vitamins A, C and B12, beta-carotene*

GOOD FOR MOTHER: *fertility, enzyme production, hormonal function, fluid retention, diabetes, maintaining blood sugar levels, high blood pressure, constipation, fatigue*

GOOD FOR BABY: *development of brain and central nervous system, cell growth and strong cell structure, healthy skin, hair and eyes, manufacture of genetic material, hard bones and teeth*

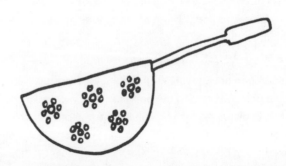

Snapper Pie

Fish is an essential part of the pregnancy diet and fabulous brain food for both you and your baby. Aim to eat fish 2 to 3 times a week. The creamy leek sauce in this pie softens the fish flavour, making it more tolerable for those experiencing food aversions. I hope this wholesome meal becomes one of your favourites.

200 g (7 oz) fresh snapper fillets,
   diced into 3-cm (1¼-inch) cubes

1 medium sweet potato, diced

2 tbs olive oil

1 leek, finely sliced

2 celery stalks, finely sliced

1 cup baby spinach leaves, finely sliced

2 bay leaves

2 tsp dried thyme

8 sheets frozen filo pastry, thawed

½ cup wheatgerm

1 egg white

white sauce:

2 tbs butter

2 tbs plain flour

1½ cups low-fat milk

1 tsp lemon rind

cracked black pepper

Preheat the oven to 200°C/400°F. Line a baking tray with baking paper.

Bring a medium saucepan of water to the boil. Add the sweet potato and cook for 10 minutes or until just tender. Drain and set aside.

Heat the oil in a heavy-based frying pan over medium heat. Cook leeks and celery until softened (approximately 3–4 minutes). Remove from heat and season with herbs and black pepper. Add sweet potato to leek mixture, mix through and set aside.

Prepare the sauce by gently melting the butter over medium heat. Reduce to a low heat. Use a wooden spoon and while stirring, add the flour. Stir continuously to remove all lumps and form a smooth paste. Gradually add milk, still stirring, until all milk is added and the sauce thickens. This may take a couple of minutes. The sauce will eventually thicken. Do not allow to boil as this may result in a lumpy sauce. Stir through lemon rind and season with black pepper. Add the white sauce to the leek and sweet potato mixture, together with the diced raw fish and baby spinach leaves. Set aside.

To make two fish parcels, each with four sheets of filo, lay one filo sheet on a clean bench top or chopping board and brush with a little olive oil. Sprinkle lightly with a little wheatgerm and lay next pastry sheet on top. Repeat this two more times, leaving the top filo sheet undressed. Set aside and repeat to prepare the remaining parcel.

Place half of the fish mixture on a diagonal across the centre of the layered pastry, leaving 5 cm at each end. Lightly whisk the egg white and brush around the edges of the pastry. Fold the pastry corner closest to you over the fish, then do the same with the two side corners and finish with the corner farthest away from you, to get an envelope effect. Seal all edges with the egg white and baste the top of each parcel with remaining egg white.

Place fish parcels on a baking tray and cook for 20 minutes, or until pastry is golden brown. Serve with steamed greens or a rocket and asparagus salad.

tip *Mussels can be added to make this a sensational seafood pie. Add 185 g (6½ oz) of canned mussels, or pre-cook fresh mussels and remove from shells. Add to recipe when you add the fish.*

GOOD SOURCE OF: *omega 3, protein, zinc, calcium, folate, vitamins A, C and B-group, magnesium, potassium, phosphorus*

GOOD FOR MOTHER: *fatigue, skin elasticity, stretch marks, toning and nourishing uterus, fluid retention, food aversions, dental problems, diabetes, calcium absorption, supporting foetal growth*

GOOD FOR BABY: *development of brain, nervous and immune systems, formation of genetic material and healthy cells, skin, hair and body fat, good eyesight, hard bones*

Ginger Salmon Curry

All the flavours of a decadent Asian curry are created in next to no time with this quick and easy curry. It contains the key essential nutrients for pregnancy, combined with the healing and therapeutic properties of ginger and garlic.

1 medium sweet potato, diced into
  2-cm (¾-inch) pieces

400 g (14 oz) salmon fillet, diced into
  3-cm (1¼-inch) cubes

1 tbs olive oil

1 x 400 g (14 oz) can tomatoes
  (salt reduced)

100 g (3½ oz) green beans, cut into
  2-cm (¾-inch) lengths

100 g (3½ oz) broccoli, cut into bite-sized florets

fresh coriander leaves to serve

curry paste:

3 tbs finely grated ginger

2 cloves garlic, roughly chopped

2 sprigs coriander, roots and stems

2 tbs finely sliced lemongrass,
  white part only

1 shallot, finely sliced

1–2 tsp red chilli, seeds and pith
  removed, chopped

71

Bring a pot of water to the boil. Add sweet potato and cook for 5 minutes, or until tender. Drain.

Make curry paste by placing all ingredients into a mortar and pestle and pound into a chunky paste or process in a food processor. Toss cubed fish through paste, coat evenly.

Heat oil in a large, non-stick frying pan over a medium heat. Add fish and quickly sear on all sides. Add tomatoes and gently stir through. Add sweet potato, beans and broccoli and mix to coat all ingredients with the curry flavours. Cover the pan and simmer for 5 minutes. Serve immediately with generous amounts of fresh coriander leaves.

GOOD SOURCE OF: *omega 3, iodine, protein, essential fatty acids, vitamins A, C and B-group including folate*

GOOD FOR MOTHER: *production of red blood cells, nausea, immune system, skin elasticity, circulation, stimulating appetite, healthy uterus, fatigue, healing properties*

GOOD FOR BABY: *development of brain, spine and central nervous system, genetic material and eyes, cell growth, formation of skin, hair and ears*

steamed Asian fish

Asian greens, fish and fresh herbs are all pregnancy superfoods, enhanced here by sensational spices for both flavour and nutritional benefits. Steaming fish is such a healthy method of cooking. All the goodness is retained in the juices, making this dish a real winner. It never fails to impress dinner guests.

2 x 150 g (5 oz) firm, thick, white

    fish fillets (barramundi or blue-eye cod)

1 bunch choy sum or bok choy

1 sprig fresh coriander (leaves for serving,

    roots for marinade)

marinade:

2 tsp finely grated fresh ginger (3-cm/1¼-inch piece)

1 clove garlic, finely grated

½–1 tsp red chilli, finely sliced lengthways

2 shallots, finely sliced into 5-cm (2-inch) lengths

100 ml rice wine vinegar

2 tbs tamari (or salt-reduced soy sauce)

1 tbs fresh lime juice

1 coriander root, thoroughly rinsed and finely chopped

2 tsp honey

Place all marinade ingredients into a medium bowl and mix to combine. Add fish fillets and marinate for 15–20 minutes.

Thoroughly rinse Asian greens and pat dry. Depending on what vegetables you are using, chop choy sum into 5-cm (2-inch) pieces (stalks and leaves) or separate individual bok choy leaves.

Half fill a wok or large saucepan with water. Sit a bamboo steamer over the wok/saucepan, ensuring the water does not touch the steamer. Water rises slightly when boiling and it is important fish parcels do not come into contact with water.

Cut two large sheets of aluminium foil (the length will need to be two and a half times the length of your fish fillet). Spread the foil flat on your kitchen bench. Cut two smaller pieces of baking paper that are slightly larger than the fish fillet. Position the paper in the centre of the foil. Fold up a 2-cm (¾-inch) edge of the baking paper on each side to form a little dish the same size as the fish fillet. This will prevent the marinade from running out on to the foil. Place each fish fillet in the baking paper cases.

Fold the edges in closer to the fillet if needed. Pour the marinade evenly over each fillet. To make the parcels, fold the two longest lengths of foil towards the centre so the edges meet in the middle above the fish. Join the edges and fold together tightly. Continue tightly folding and rolling down the foil until you reach the fillet. Fold the remaining edges in to also meet in the middle and again fold tightly and roll down towards the fillet to create a neat parcel. It is important to tightly seal and secure all sides to prevent the marinade and cooking juices seeping out during cooking. Repeat method for remaining fish fillet.

Bring the water in the wok to the boil. Place fish parcels in the steamer, cover and steam for 10–15 minutes. The flesh of fish turns opaque in colour when cooked and flakes easily with a fork. Towards the end of cooking, toss choy sum in the steamer and steam for 1–2 minutes. Open the parcels and serve on rice, together with the choy sum. Pour cooking juices over the dish and finish with fresh coriander on top.

73

tip *If you find making the parcels too involved, place a sheet of baking paper in the steamer and steam the fillets unmarinated. Gently heat the ginger and soy marinade in a saucepan and drizzle over the cooked fish and vegetables.*

GOOD SOURCE OF: *omega 3, protein, zinc, calcium, vitamins A, C and B-group including folate, magnesium, potassium, phosphorus, antioxidants, fibre*

GOOD FOR MOTHER: *building protein stores, toning and nourishing the uterus, skin elasticity, fatigue, nourishing heart and other major organs, boosting immunity*

GOOD FOR BABY: *reducing risk of birth defects, development of brain, spine, immune and central nervous systems, growth of healthy skin, hair and ears, eyesight, strong bones, production of blood and body cells*

Steamed Chicken in a Delicate Ginger and Lemon Broth

This delicately flavoured chicken tastes so nourishing and cleansing you just know it is doing wonders for your health. It is a fabulous tonic for general wellbeing. The combination of ingredients promotes healthy blood circulation, calms the digestive tract, wards off nausea and boosts the immune system. This is also excellent for food aversions as the broth alone is an easily digestible source of protein and goodness. Although this is a first trimester recipe, I recommend eating it throughout your entire pregnancy and beyond.

5-cm (2-inch) piece fresh ginger

1 large eggplant, diced into 2-cm (¾-inch) cubes

1 red onion, diced

1 x 1.6 kg (3.2 lb) organic/chemical-free whole chicken

2 lemons

2 tsp olive oil

cracked black pepper

small pinch of iodised (table) salt

noodles (soba, rice or egg)

1 bunch boy choy or broccoli

You will need a large steamer with insert steamer basket for this recipe. Fill the steamer to just below the steamer basket level.

Finely slice 1 tablespoon of the fresh ginger and cut the remaining ginger into small chunks.

Prepare eggplant and onion and combine with the finely sliced ginger. Mix together and spread this over the base of the steamer basket but avoid spreading too close to the edges of the basket.

Rinse chicken inside and out and trim any excess fat from around the neck. Pat dry with a paper towel. Cut one of the lemons into quarters. Insert the quarters and remaining ginger pieces into the cavity of the chicken. Place the chicken on top of the eggplant mixture and squeeze the juice of half a lemon over the chicken, along with the 2 teaspoons of olive oil. Season generously with black pepper and a small pinch of salt.

Cover the steamer with a lid and bring the water to the boil. Reduce to a simmer and steam chicken for 50–60 minutes, or until cooked through. Check your water level once or twice during cooking and top up if necessary.

In the meantime, cook noodles as per packet directions and prepare vegetables.

Once the chicken is cooked, lift the steamer tray with cooked chicken dish out of the steamer and put to one side on a plate to drain any excess juices.

The water in the bottom of the steamer has combined with the cooking juices and become a delicious and nourishing broth. Strain it through a sieve and then return to the pan. Simmer for 3–5 minutes to reduce slightly. You could even cook your noodles in the broth.

Meanwhile, lightly steam the vegetables and remove the white meat from the chicken and shred or cut into thin slices. Discard the skin or fatty tissue of the chicken.

75

Divide the noodles evenly between two bowls. Top with the eggplant mixture, followed by the chicken. Pour the broth over the chicken and finish with the steamed greens.

Serve with freshly cracked black pepper and squeezed lemon as desired.

GOOD SOURCE OF: *protein, iron, vitamins B3, B5, B6 and B12, folate, selenium, phosphorus, potassium, zinc, fibre*

GOOD FOR MOTHER: *fatigue, nausea, colds and flu, immunity, cleansing digestive system, food aversions, circulation, production of red blood cells, healthy skin and hair, hormonal function*

GOOD FOR BABY: *development of brain, skin, hair, ears, eyes and central nervous system, cell production*

Moroccan Lamb and Lentils

Moroccan cuisine is extremely healthy, mainly due to its heavy use of spices. Spices minimise the need to use fat or sugar to flavour and tenderise food. They also have therapeutic qualities, aiding digestion, circulation and nausea. Lamb is a fantastic protein and iron source. It is important to begin pregnancy with healthy levels of both of these nutrients for healthy blood, foetal growth and to avoid anaemia and fatigue. This marinated lamb is so versatile and can be used in many different dishes and should be enjoyed throughout all three trimesters.

400 g (14 oz) lean lamb fillets

Moroccan marinade:

1 tsp cumin

1 tsp coriander

1 tsp paprika

1 garlic clove, crushed

1 tbs fresh mint, chopped

1 tbs lemon juice

1 tbs olive oil

lentil dish:

½ cup lentils (Du Puy, or French green lentils, or canned lentils)

2 shallots, finely diced

½ medium red capsicum, finely diced

½ cup fresh coriander

cracked black pepper

small pinch ground cumin

flaxseed oil, to serve

large handful spinach leaves, shredded

low-fat plain yoghurt to serve

Combine all marinade ingredients in a bowl. Thoroughly mix to form a paste. Trim the lamb fillets of any visible fat. Score shallow, diagonal lines across the lamb and generously coat the fillets with the paste. Allow to marinate for 20–30 minutes, or longer if time allows.

Meanwhile, prepare the lentil dish. Place 3 cups of water in a medium to large saucepan and bring to the boil. Rinse lentils with clean water through a strainer. Place lentils in saucepan and cook for 10–15 minutes. Be sure not to overcook as lentils will lose their texture and turn mushy. If using canned lentils, strain and rinse thoroughly.

Prepare remaining vegetables for the lentil dish. Drain lentils and return to saucepan. Add shallots, capsicum and coriander. Season with black pepper and a pinch of cumin. Cover the saucepan with a lid to keep warm.

Cook the lamb on a preheated grill for approximately 5 minutes on each side, depending on the thickness of the fillet. Transfer lamb to a plate, cover with foil and rest for 5 minutes. Resting meat allows the cooking juices to settle. If you slice meat immediately after cooking, these juices often escape, leaving the meat tough and dry.

Drizzle the flaxseed oil over the lentils and gently toss through. Evenly divide the lentils and arrange in the middle of each serving plate. Top with the shredded spinach.

Slice lamb fillets on the diagonal and place on top of the spinach and finish with a generous dollop of yoghurt to serve and a little black pepper.

tip *Serve lamb fillets with a herbed yoghurt sauce and a mixed leaf salad or combine sliced fillets in a wrap with hummus, tomato and fresh coriander, parsley or baby spinach leaves. Alternatively, cube uncooked marinated lamb and thread onto skewers. Cook on a barbeque and serve on a bed of white bean puree and steamed greens. For a complete vegetarian protein option, add a cup of basmati rice to the lentil dish and serve with yoghurt.*

77

GOOD SOURCE OF: *protein, vitamins A, C, B12 and B6, iron, selenium, zinc, folate, phosphorus, fibre, low GI carbohydrate, magnesium, calcium, essential fatty acids*

GOOD FOR MOTHER: *digestion, circulation, fatigue, diabetes, nausea, converting food to fuel, anaemia, constipation, production of red blood cells for both mother and baby*

GOOD FOR BABY: *manufacture of genetic material, development of baby's brain, nervous system, growth of all major organs, skin, hair, ears and eyes*

Barbeque Lamb fillets with Mushy Peas

Chances are this recipe will become a favourite. It is *so* quick and easy to prepare and is a perfect example of eating enough nutrients for two. It is not a stretch to say that this is a completely balanced meal. You might be surprised to learn that lamb actually contains more iron than beef. And the pea belongs to the legume family and is incredibly nutrient rich. It contains eight vitamins, plus minerals and loads of dietary fibre. Peas have a low GI rating to help maintain blood sugar levels and reduce the risk of developing many of the common complaints of pregnancy, especially nausea and fatigue.

400 g (14 oz) lean lamb fillets

olive oil for basting

lots of cracked black pepper

400 g (14 oz) frozen peas

2 tbs fresh mint

2 tbs low-fat plain yoghurt

2 tsp olive oil

Preheat barbeque or grill to a medium heat. Trim lamb of any excess fat and lightly baste with olive oil and season with black pepper. Place the lamb on the barbeque or grill and cook for 4 minutes on each side, or until cooked. Set aside in a warm place and let lamb rest for a couple of minutes before serving.

While the lamb is cooking, add the peas to boiling water and cook for 2–3 minutes. Drain and put the peas into a food processor, together with the mint and yoghurt. Process for a minute or two, scrape the peas from the side, add the olive oil, and process for a further minute or so until you have a puree consistency. I like to have a few chunky peas in mine. Season generously with black pepper.

Place a large dollop of the peas on the centre of each plate and top with the lamb fillets.

tip *Serve with baked parsnips or Doongara rice on the side. Doongara rice (clever rice) can be found in most supermarkets and has a low GI rating.*

GOOD SOURCE OF: *protein, iron, vitamins A, C, K and B-group, especially B6 and B12, folate, selenium, zinc, potassium, phosphorus, calcium, magnesium, fibre, essential fatty acids*

GOOD FOR MOTHER: *fatigue, hypertension, converting food to fuel, constipation, healthy heart and blood, immunity, diabetes, blood sugar levels, increasing blood supply, anaemia*

GOOD FOR BABY: *reducing risk of birth defects, providing building blocks for normal growth, cell production, brain and nervous system, eyesight, initial heartbeat and blood circulation*

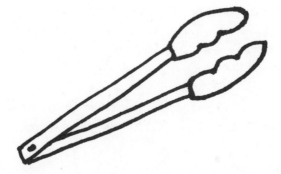

Beef Pasta with Almond and Avocado Pesto

This recipe has been devised to assist with food aversions to protein, a common first trimester complaint. The use of avocado and almonds in my healthy version of pesto creates a sublime, creamy pasta dish that almost disguises the flavour of the beef. I have included vitamin C-rich tomatoes and broccoli to maximise the absorption of iron. Every mouthful of this meal counts.

2 cups Soyaroni pasta

200g (7 oz) lean rump steak

1 punnet cherry tomatoes, halved

1 cup mushrooms, quartered

2 cups broccoli, cut into small florets

cracked black pepper

avocado and almond pesto:

½ cup almonds

1 bunch fresh basil

2 tbs lemon juice

1 clove garlic, crushed

½ avocado

Heat barbeque plate or grill.

To make the pesto, place the almonds in a blender and roughly chop. Add basil and process until just combined. Add lemon juice, garlic and avocado. Briefly blend again for a slightly chunky texture.

Bring a pot of water to the boil and cook pasta according to packet directions, until just al dente. Strain, saving a little cooking water to moisten the dish if necessary. Put cooked pasta back in the saucepan and cover to keep warm.

Cook rump steak on the preheated grill or barbeque. Remove from heat and cover with foil. Meanwhile, toss tomatoes, mushroom and broccoli in a non-stick frying pan and cook for 2–3 minutes. Add to pasta.

Thinly slice the steak and add to pasta dish with a little of the reserved cooking water. Stir through the pesto and cook for one minute over a medium heat to coat and combine ingredients. Turn heat off, cover and allow the pesto to melt through the pasta. Season with black pepper.

tip *This pesto is extremely versatile. Use as a spread for sandwiches or spread a generous dollop over grilled chicken breasts and serve with a green salad for another delicious meal.*

GOOD SOURCE OF: *iron, protein, folate, vitamins A, C, K and B-group, fibre, calcium, magnesium, potassium, omega 3, complex carbohydrate*

GOOD FOR MOTHER: *fatigue, healthy blood/anaemia, nausea, food aversions, digestion, toning heart muscles, healthy skin, hair and eyes, skin elasticity, hypertension*

GOOD FOR BABY: *vital early development of brain and spine, reducing risk of birth defects, production of genetic material, major organs and muscles, proper foetal growth*

SLOW-COOKED BEEF AND VEGETABLE STEW

This dish was created to overcome food aversions to both protein and Brussels sprouts. Brussels sprouts are an important nutrient source in the pregnancy diet, but sadly not many people are partial to this humble little veg. I convinced a few anti-Brusselers to taste this dish and they loved it, not even noticing the sprouts. The delicious flavours of the spices, vegetables and stock do well to disguise the taste of the beef and sprouts. This is pure, old-fashioned comfort food that may assist with nausea and is excellent for the blood. Unfortunately, there are no shorts cuts to achieving the melt-in-the mouth tender beef we get by slowly stewing the meat. It does take some time to cook, but it is certainly worth the effort.

500 g (1 lb 2 oz) blade/chuck steak

1 tbs plain flour

1 tbs paprika

1 tbs caraway seeds, roughly ground

1 tbs ground coriander

cracked black pepper

3 tbs olive oil

2 garlic cloves, chopped

1 brown onion, thinly sliced

2 potatoes, cut into bite-sized pieces

1 carrot, chopped into bite-sized pieces

2 celery sticks, chopped into 2 cm lengths

400 g (14 oz) can of salt-reduced tomatoes

½ cup (125 ml/4 fl oz) chicken stock, boiling

200 g (7 oz) Brussels sprouts, quartered

½ cup fresh parsley, chopped

Trim the beef of excess fat. Cube the beef, slicing along and with the grain of the meat for a tender result. Cut into 3-cm (1¼-inch) cubes.

Combine flour, spices and black pepper in a bowl and mix well. Add the cubed beef and toss to evenly coat all sides. Heat 2 tablespoons of oil in a heavy-based non-stick pan. Add beef and quickly sear all sides. Remove beef from the pan and place in a bowl. Wipe the pan clean with a paper towel.

In the same pan, heat the remaining oil over a medium heat. Saute the garlic and onion for 3–5 minutes, or until onions are transparent. Turn the heat down if the garlic begins to brown. Add potatoes, carrots and celery. Mix through and coat with the onion mixture.

Return the beef and its juices to the pan, together with the tomatoes and stock, then season with black pepper. Turn the heat down to low and very slowly bring to a gentle simmer. You do not want to boil the casserole at all.

Cover and simmer for 2 hours if possible. Stir occasionally and check the casserole does not reach boiling point. Add the Brussels sprouts 15 minutes prior to the end of cooking time. If at this stage the sauce needs a little thickening, remove the lid for the last 15 minutes. If the sauce still does not thicken, add 1 tablespoon of lecithin or cornflour and stir to dissolve.

83

Remove from heat and stir through the fresh parsley. Season to taste and serve.

tip *As with all stews and casseroles, the flavour of this dish improves over time. This can be made a day ahead and is suitable for freezing. Simply follow the recipe without adding the parsley. Parsley, or any fresh herb, should be added to a dish just prior to serving for maximum nutrition. Cool casserole completely and store in an airtight container in the fridge for 2–3 days, or freeze for up to 2–3 months.*

GOOD SOURCE OF: *iron, protein, zinc, carbohydrates, folate, B-group vitamins, calcium, beta-carotene*

GOOD FOR MOTHER: *food aversions, fatigue, anaemia, healthy heart, blood and skin, increasing blood supply*

GOOD FOR BABY: *manufacture of genetic material, healthy cell growth, development of all major organs, strong external structures, fuelling foetal growth*

Steak and Stuffed Mushrooms

Steak and mushrooms are great mates on the plate, complementing each other's flavours. In the pregnancy diet they play a vital role in the growth and development of your baby. Both foods contain vitamin B12 and iron to promote the production of red blood cells, healthy blood and reduce the risk of anaemia. They are also absolutely essential for the development of your baby's brain and central nervous system. I've jazzed up the mushroom in this recipe with a nourishing topping, making this yet another nutritionally outstanding meal for pregnancy.

2 x 150 g (5 oz) rump or fillet steak

olive oil

cracked black pepper

2 large field mushrooms

125 g (4½ oz) cottage cheese

1 red capsicum, diced

½ small red onion, diced

2 tbs fresh basil

2 tbs fresh parsley

½ cup wheatgerm

1 tbs grated parmesan cheese

200 g steamed asparagus or broccoli to serve

Heat grill or barbeque. Trim steaks of visible fat. Lightly baste with olive oil and season with black pepper.

Preheat oven to 180°C/350°F. Line a baking tray with baking paper.

Wipe mushrooms with a paper towel to remove any excess dirt. Remove stems and place mushrooms upside down (stem side up) on the baking tray.

Combine cottage cheese, capsicum, onion and herbs and spoon into the mushroom caps.

Mix together wheatgerm and parmesan cheese and sprinkle on top of the mushroom stuffing.

Bake in the oven for 10–15 minutes. Mushrooms will soften and the topping with brown.

Meanwhile, cook steaks to your liking and a few minutes prior to serving, steam the vegetables.

tip *The stuffed mushrooms are a protein-rich meal on their own and are perfect for vegetarians or as a smaller meal.*

GOOD SOURCE OF: *iron, protein, vitamins A, B2, B12, C, D and K, calcium, phosphorus, potassium, selenium, fibre*

GOOD FOR MOTHER: *anaemia, fatigue, fertility, circulation, immunity, healthy blood supply, strong bones*

GOOD FOR BABY: *development of brain and nervous system, manufacture of genetic material, strong bons, teeth and nails, general foetal growth*

Roast Pork and Pears

Pork and pears are a delicious combination and this no-fuss meal can be ready to eat in just 30 minutes. This recipe is rich in the B-group vitamins which help with nausea and play a major role in breaking down carbohydrates and protein for energy.

½ cup (125 ml/4 fl oz) white wine vinegar

1 tsp freshly grated ginger

1 ripe pear

1 shallot

1 x 400 g (14 oz) lean pork fillet

1 tbs olive oil

1 cup frozen green peas, to serve

1 bunch fresh asparagus, to serve

6 baby new potatoes, to serve

Preheat oven to 180°C/ 350°F (fan forced oven).

Combine vinegar and grated ginger in a medium-sized bowl. Slice pear lengthways and add to bowl. Gently toss to coat.

Finely slice the shallot on a diagonal angle and set aside. Trim all visible fat from pork and cut fillet in half. Baste with olive oil and place in a shallow baking dish. Sprinkle shallots over the fillet and pour over the pear mixture. Cover baking dish with foil and bake for 15–20 minutes. The small amount of alcohol present in the vinegar dissipates during cooking.

Serve with the green peas, steamed asparagus and new potatoes.

GOOD SOURCE OF: *protein, vitamins A, C, K and B-group, especially B1, B3 and folate, potassium, fibre*

GOOD FOR MOTHER: *nausea, digestion, fatigue, circulation, hypertension, loss of appetite, heart function, strengthening blood vessels, immunity*

GOOD FOR BABY: *proper development of neural tube and central nervous system, production of haemoglobin, formation of skin, hair and eyes, supporting foetal growth*

Chickpea and Vegetable Curry

Yum! This curry is a fantastic way to enjoy the unbeatable goodness of chickpeas and dose up on your vegetable intake. It is a great protein and carbohydrate source for energy and to fuel foetal growth. As with all curries, flavours improve over time, making this an ideal work lunch. Make a pot on the weekend and take individual servings to heat up at work. This recipe is a complete protein option for vegetarians when eaten with basmati rice.

½ tsp ground cumin

1 tsp ground coriander

1 cinnamon stick, snapped in half

⅛ tsp ground turmeric

½ tsp paprika

2 garlic cloves, finely grated

2 tsp fresh ginger, finely grated

1 tbs olive oil

1 small brown onion, diced

4 tomatoes, diced

200 g (7 oz) cooked chickpeas, or 400 g (14 oz) can once drained

1 medium sweet potato, diced

1 cup (250ml/ 8 fl oz) stock

150 g (5 oz) green beans, diced

200 g (7 oz) cauliflower, cut into bite-sized florets

1 cup baby spinach leaves

250 g (9 oz) low-fat cottage cheese

½ cup fresh coriander

Combine spices, garlic and ginger in a small saucer. Heat olive oil in a large saucepan. Cook spices for 1–2 minutes until aromatic. Add onion and cook for 2–3 minutes or until transparent, stirring constantly. Add diced tomatoes. Reduce heat, cover and simmer for 5 minutes, stirring occasionally to prevent sticking. Add chickpeas, sweet potato and the stock. Combine and coat all ingredients with the spiced tomatoes. Cover and simmer for 15 minutes. Add beans and cauliflower, cover and cook for a further 10 minutes. Turn the heat off. If you are pre-making or freezing this dish, finish recipe here and proceed with recipe just prior to serving.

To serve, stir the spinach leaves and cottage cheese through the curry. Cover and allow the heat to slightly wilt the leaves and melt the cheese. Stir through fresh coriander and serve with basmati rice. Serves 4.

tip *Yoghurt could be used as a substitute for the cottage cheese.*

GOOD SOURCE OF: *protein, fibre, iron, calcium, magnesium, phosphorus, B-group vitamins including folate, beta-carotene, zinc, complex carbohydrates*

GOOD FOR MOTHER: *vegetarians, constipation, digestion, fatigue, hypertension, diabetes*

GOOD FOR BABY: *healthy blood and skin, strong bones, cell growth, formation of skin, bones and eyes, reducing risk of birth defects, fuelling foetal growth, development of nervous system, all major organs and limbs*

Blackeye Bean and Broccoli Salad

This salad packs a nutritional punch and is fantastic for preconception and the first trimester. It is very rich in folate and also boasts vital minerals such as zinc, selenium and calcium. It is a complete vegetarian protein source when combined with wild or brown rice, or a wonderful accompaniment to any grilled meat. For a quick version, tinned mixed beans can be used in place of the blackeye beans.

½ cup raw black eyed beans	**lemon soy dressing:**
½ cup brown/wild rice	2 tbs lemon juice
½ cup almonds	1 tsp tamari
200 g (7 oz) broccoli	2 tbs flaxseed or extra virgin olive oil
⅓ cup parsley, finely chopped	½ clove garlic
2 spring onions, finely sliced	pinch cracked black pepper

Rinse black eyed beans and place in a medium saucepan with 3–4 cups of water. Bring to the boil and cook for 25 minutes, or until tender. Be careful not to overcook the beans as they will turn mushy and unappealing. You can also soak beans to reduce cooking time (see Tip).

Cook rice according to packet directions. Roast almonds in a moderate oven for 5 minutes. Wash and trim broccoli into 2 cm pieces and lightly steam for 2–3 minutes.

Prepare remaining salad ingredients and combine in a salad bowl. Combine dressing ingredients in a small cup or jar and whisk or shake vigorously.

Rinse beans and add to salad bowl with cooked rice and broccoli. Pour over dressing and toss.

 Black eyed beans are an excellent source of folate, selenium and fibre. They are available from all good health food stores in their dried form, but not so readily available in a can. Many people shy away from cooking legumes, but it really is a great habit to get into as they are preservative free and very economical. You do have to plan ahead and soak the beans. I usually toss them into a saucepan filled with plenty of water in the morning and by the evening they are ready to cook. Black eyed beans require minimum preparation time, with 2–3 hours of soaking and only 10 minutes cooking time.

GOOD SOURCE OF: *protein, folate, selenium, calcium, zinc, magnesium, potassium, phosphorus, vitamins C, E, K and B-group, fibre*

GOOD FOR MOTHER: *reproduction, excellent energy source, circulation, constipation, immunity, digestion*

GOOD FOR BABY: *development of neural tube, brain and major organs, production of DNA, cell growth, healthy blood, growth of muscles, skin, hair, eyes, strong bones*

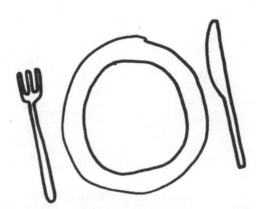

Berry Baked Custards

All the goodness of eggs, yoghurt and berries—pregnancy superfoods—are combined to create this delicious dessert. It is another perfect example of eating the nutrients for two and is a great way to start your pregnancy. Our baked berry custards can be served warm, straight from the oven, or are just as yummy chilled for a protein/calcium-rich snack.

> 200 g (7 oz) fresh blueberries, or if frozen, completely thawed
>
> 4 eggs
>
> 1 tbs self-raising flour
>
> 1 tsp vanilla essence
>
> 1 cup low-fat plain yoghurt
>
> 1 tbs honey

Preheat oven to 180°C/350°F. You can prepare this dish as individual servings in four small ramekins, or in a 20-cm (8-inch) baking dish. Cooking times will vary as indicated below.

If you are using frozen berries, place in a sieve and drain excess juice. Drain over a small bowl or cup and drink the juice! It's good for you.

Beat eggs until light and fluffy. Add flour and vanilla essence and beat for 30 seconds.

Pour yoghurt and honey in a bowl (or directly into the baking dish if using) and stir to combine. Add the egg mixture and lightly whisk together. Gently stir through berries and the mixture is ready to bake. If using ramekins, pour equal amounts of the mixture into each ramekin. The mixture should fill approximately three-quarters of each.

The baking dish will take 30 minutes to cook; individual ramekins 15 minutes. Remove from oven and cool slightly before serving with a dollop of yoghurt if desired.

91

GOOD SOURCE OF: *protein, zinc, iodine, iron, omega 3, vitamins A, C, D and B-group including B12, selenium, phosphorus, potassium, magnesium, calcium*

GOOD FOR MOTHER: *digestion, nausea, food aversion, calcium absorption, strengthening blood capillaries, brain function, diabetes*

GOOD FOR BABY: *healthy heart, kidney and liver, strong bones, teeth and nails, normal foetal growth, development of brain and central nervous system, eyesight*

Spiced Poached Pears

Poached pears never fail to impress, which astounds me considering how easy they are to make. This is my pregnant version of the classic dish, poached pears in red wine, using non-alcoholic sparkling grape juice—the choice to cook with wine during your pregnancy is a personal one.

2 large firm pears (look for pears with a flat base)

3 cups (750 ml/24 fl oz) sparkling red grape juice

1 vanilla bean, split lengthways

2 star anise

2 cinnamon sticks

5 cloves

low-fat yoghurt to serve

Peel pears, leaving stem and core intact. Pour grape juice into a medium, heavy-based saucepan. Split vanilla bean lengthways but do not scrape out seeds—they will come out naturally during cooking. Add vanilla and all remaining spices to grape juice.

Place pears in the saucepan. Bring the poaching liquid to the boil and then reduce to a simmer. Cover and poach. Cooking time can be as little as 20 minutes, or as long as one hour. Obviously, the longer you cook the pears the more time they will have to absorb the wonderful flavours. If you do have an hour to spare, cook the pears on a very low heat. Otherwise, 20 minutes is absolutely fine on a medium simmer. Serve with vanilla or plain yoghurt.

tip *Traditional recipes stand the pears on their bases for the full cooking time. I like my pears to evenly take on the colour of the poaching liquid and so lay them on their side, gently rotating at 10 minute intervals. If cooking for one hour, I stand the pears on their base for the last 20 minutes.*

GOOD SOURCE OF: *fibre, potassium, vitamins A, C and B12, calcium, protein*

GOOD FOR MOTHER: *cleansing, calming and healing the digestive system, circulation, constipation*

GOOD FOR BABY: *formation of healthy skin, hair, eyes, ears and external structures, nervous system*

fruit Creams

Bananas are nature's fast food. They are packaged, portable and loaded with nourishment. This recipe takes the banana one step further to make the most of its creamy, robust texture by freezing it to produce a delicious dessert. Berries are another pregnancy superfood and one of the best antioxidant food sources you can eat. The combination of the two makes this an incredibly healthy, dairy-free dessert. You will need to pre-plan this recipe as the fruit must be frozen overnight.

3 large bananas

1 cup frozen blueberries, or forest fruit berries

Peel bananas, wrap tightly in cling wrap and place in the freezer overnight.

To prepare, remove bananas and berries from freezer and allow to soften at room temperature for 20 minutes. Roughly chop the bananas, then place all of the fruit in a food processor and blend until thick and creamy.

Scoop into serving glasses and eat immediately. This dessert will go runny, like ice-cream, if left at room temperature for a long period. Serves 2 to 4.

93

tip *Once fully prepared, this dessert can be frozen. Remove from freezer 15 to 20 minutes prior to eating to allow it to soften a little.*

GOOD SOURCE OF: *potassium, folate, vitamins B, C and E, fibre, antioxidants*

GOOD FOR MOTHER: *dairy-free diets, protecting against cell damage, strengthening blood capillaries, varicose veins, immune system, healthy kidneys, skin, teeth and gums, constipation*

GOOD FOR BABY: *reducing risk of birth defects, formation of eyes, general foetal growth*

fresh fruit Crumbles

Crumbles are a quick and easy dessert and our oat-based topping makes this a healthy version. For a true crumble we use a little pure butter rather than margarine. It is a natural product and contains useful nutrients such as vitamins A, D and E, which are fabulous for the skin and the eyes.

I have provided two fruit filling options for you to choose from: classic apple and berry, which is bursting with antioxidants for excellent health and immunity, and the heavenly pear and banana which promotes a healthy digestive tract and helps retain calcium in the bones.

Apple and Berry fruit Crumble

½ cup (125 ml/4 fl oz) water

½ tsp vanilla essence

½ tsp cinnamon

2 apples, diced with skin on
  (granny smiths or pink lady
  varieties work well)

1 cup frozen mixed berries,
  defrosted

Crumble:

1 cup rolled oats or rolled barley

1/3 cup almonds or hazelnuts

½ cup wheatgerm

1 tsp cinnamon

20 g (¾ oz) unsalted butter, melted

1 tbs grape seed or olive oil

1 tsp honey

low-fat yoghurt to serve

Preheat oven to 180°C/350°F. I like to cook the berry crumbles in individual ramekins, but a medium baking dish is also fine to use.

To make the crumble, place oats, nuts, wheatgerm and cinnamon into a food processor and process into fine crumbs. Pour the melted butter, oil and honey in a small cup and whisk to combine and dissolve the honey. Pour over the oat mixture and mix through.

Combine water, vanilla and cinnamon in a medium bowl. Add diced apple and berries and mix through. Scatter evenly over the base of the baking dish or divide evenly among the ramekins.

Sprinkle crumble evenly over the top of the fruit and bake for 20–25 minutes, or until crumble is golden brown.

Serve with a generous dollop of yoghurt for a boost of calcium.

94

GOOD SOURCE OF: *vitamins A, C, D, E and B-group, calcium, fibre, antioxidants, zinc, protein, omega 3*

GOOD FOR MOTHER: *fatigue, fertility, immunity, diabetes, healthy skin, hair and eyes, hypertension, kidney function, strengthening blood capillaries, protecting body cells*

GOOD FOR BABY: *fuelling foetal growth, development of all major organs and central nervous system, heartbeat and blood circulation, strong healthy bone and cell structure, eyesight*

Pear and Banana Fruit Crumble

1 pear, diced with skin on

2 bananas, peeled and cut
   on diagonal in long slices

1 tbs fresh lemon juice

Crumble:

1 cup rolled oats or rolled barley

⅓ cup almonds or hazelnuts

½ cup wheatgerm

1 tsp cinnamon

20 g (¾ oz) unsalted butter, melted

1 tbs grape seed or olive oil

1 tsp honey

low-fat yoghurt to serve

Preheat oven to 170°C/330°F. Make crumble as per previous recipe.

Place fruit in a medium-sized baking dish. Drizzle over lemon juice and mix through to coat the fruit. Sprinkle the crumble evenly over the bananas and pears and bake for 20–25 minutes, or until the crumble is golden brown.

Serve with a generous dollop of yoghurt for a boost of calcium.

GOOD SOURCE OF: *vitamins A, D, E and B-group, calcium, magnesium, potassium, fibre, omega 3, zinc, protein*

GOOD FOR MOTHER: *fatigue, digestion, reflux, diabetes, healthy heart, skin, hair and eyes, hypertension, fertility, leg cramps, calcium absorption*

GOOD FOR BABY: *development of all major organs and central nervous system, first heartbeat and blood circulation, strong healthy bone and cell structure, eyesight*

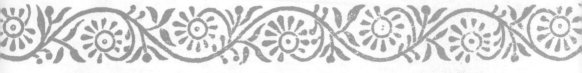

❀ second trimester weeks 14 to 28

This is the most comfortable and enjoyable trimester. You will probably feel and look fabulous. The majority of the symptoms of the first trimester should subside and energy levels return. Exercise is another necessity for a healthy pregnancy, so enjoy making good use of this energy.

Many women notice they 'glow' during the second trimester. This is attributable to hormonal activity, increased metabolic rate and blood volume. More blood is pumping around the body, so it is closer to the skin, hence the glow.

But don't be fooled—your body is working harder than ever to maintain the pregnancy and your growing baby. Continue to nourish your body wisely, eat regularly and do not skip meals. Calcium is especially important during the second trimester, with daily requirements almost doubling. The main complaints of the second trimester are constipation, heartburn, reflux and bleeding gums.

The essential nutrients needed at this time are: calcium (need to double intake), iron, essential fatty acids (vitamin E), vitamin C, B-group vitamins (folate, B1, B2, B3, B12), omega 3, iodine, magnesium.

PROGRESSION OF BABY

WHAT'S HAPPENING	WHAT'S NEEDED
Fully formed (except lungs), with structures now maturing	
Everything growing rapidly, including brain, muscles, skin and hair. Fat begins to form	zinc, calcium, magnesium, protein, vitamins C, A and B2, selenium
Bones hardened by 16 weeks	calcium, vitamins C and D, magnesium
Muscles and nerves connect and respond to the brain	calcium, magnesium, potassium vitamins B5 and B6
Brain, nervous and immune systems develop	omega 3, zinc, iodine, calcium, vitamin B6

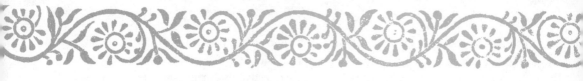

PROGRESSION OF MOTHER

WHAT'S HAPPENING	WHAT'S NEEDED
Appetite returns, food aversions subside Acute sense of smell. Change to the palate	
Blood volume still increasing. Susceptible to anaemia	protein, iron, folate, vitamins B12 and B5
Immune system vulnerable	zinc, essential fatty acids, vitamins C and A
Dental problems—bleeding gums	calcium, vitamin C

Common complaints of the second trimester

Anaemia

Anaemia is very common in pregnancy. It is usually diagnosed between weeks 20 to 28 as a result of an increase in the mother's blood volume, which peaks during this time. Extra blood is needed during pregnancy by the uterus, breasts and other organs and to prepare for blood loss during delivery. As volume increases it becomes more diluted and the need for more haemoglobin arises. Haemoglobin transports oxygen around the body via the red blood cells.

The volume of blood will increase regardless of your nutritional intake. It is the red blood cell count that is of concern. Red blood cells of a healthy woman with adequate iron levels will multiply at a consistent and proportionate rate. Those of an under-nourished woman will not.

Anaemia is a shortage of haemoglobin in the blood that equates to low levels of oxygen in body cells and vital organs. Prolonged effects can weaken the body's immune system and resistance to infections, or induce heart attacks and angina. Deficient or low levels of iron, folate or vitamin B12 can trigger anaemia. Symptoms include fatigue, shortness of breath, heart palpitations, chest pains, pale skin, headaches and leg cramps.

While both iron and folate should play a main part in your diet from as early as preconception, it is absolutely essential your iron intake is maintained during the next (third) trimester. If healthy levels of iron and vitamin B12 are maintained throughout your pregnancy you won't run the risk of developing anaemia. Treatment usually requires taking supplements that can have side effects, including constipation, which is already exacerbated towards end of term. A varied diet should ensure you do not become deficient in any nutrient throughout your pregnancy.

A baby can never be born anaemic, but an anaemic mother runs a high risk of suffering the effects of profound anaemia for the rest of her life. Women lose a lot of blood during childbirth—up to 500 millilitres (16 fluid ounces), and if haemoglobin levels are too low, a blood transfusion may be necessary. Tiredness and fatigue are symptoms of anaemia and this is certainly not the best way to enjoy the first few months of your new baby.

Tips to avoid anaemia include:

- eat foods rich in iron and folate—lean meats, parsley, green leafy vegetables, wholegrains, dried apricots and beetroot
- eat these foods with vitamin C sources to maximise absorption
- monitor blood levels with regular check-ups, as advised by your health practitioner
- increase iron intake towards end of second trimester and during third.

Digestive Problems

Reflux, heartburn and indigestion affect at least 50 percent of women during their pregnancy. Digestive problems may develop during the second trimester, but are likely to be more exacerbated during the third due to the pressure of the growing baby on the stomach.

Increased hormone levels are the main cause of digestive problems. They relax the stomach muscles, which causes food to pass through the digestive tract more slowly. This makes stomach acids rise to the oesophagus, promoting reflux or heartburn. Food sitting in the stomach can also trigger bloating and indigestion. Overweight women are more inclined to suffer from digestive problems as the excess weight puts additional pressure on an already squished tummy.

Digestion problems are very individual, but general tips for avoiding them include:

- eat smaller, more frequent meals and nutritional snacks
- eat food slowly
- drink lots of fluids between meals, but never with meals
- sit upright when eating and don't lie down for at least two hours after a meal
- take a slow walk after each meal

- drink a glass of milk before sleeping to neutralise stomach acids—cold milk can ease heartburn, while warm milk can induce a restful sleep
- drink a cup of chamomile tea before bed
- increase dietary intake of the B-complex vitamins
- eat raw vegetables and salads with meals to aid digestion
- avoid the following foods, which are known to stimulate heartburn:
  - fried, fatty or acidic foods
  - hot, spicy or heavily seasoned foods
  - tomato-based products
  - citrus fruits and juices
  - cheese just prior to bedtime
  - peppermint—peppermint tea is good for digestion but is not a remedy for reflux
  - vinegar, chocolate, carbonated drinks, tea and coffee.

Foods that aid digestion include:

99

- bitter foods, such as rocket and watercress are excellent digestive aids
- mint in all forms—use fresh mint in salads, salsas and desserts or dried peppermint and spearmint tea
- fennel—infuse seeds in boiling water as tea, or use as a spice in cooking
- ginger—use fresh slices in tea, juices and stir fries, or as a spice in cooking
- cumin, cardamom, turmeric and caraway spices
- banana, apple, pineapple, papaya, paw paw, tomato, carrot and celery
- chamomile tea
- milk and yoghurt are said to be useful for reflux.

Constipation

Constipation is more common during the second and third trimesters, but can be experienced as early as the first trimester, so it is advisable to eat fibre-rich foods from as early as possible. These foods are usually highly nutritious and are welcome additions to the diet. Constipation is known to continue after delivery, so be advised keep up the fibre well into post-partum.

Drinking lots of water is important in relieving constipation. If fluid is not increased with fibre, the problem can actually worsen. Fluids keep the bowel lubricated and prevent fibre from bulking and blocking up the digestive tract. Drink *at least* eight glasses per day. Coffee, tea and soft drinks don't count as they are diuretics and can actually dehydrate you. Freshly squeezed juices are your next best alternative to water.

Constipation in pregnancy can be caused by hormonal changes, the pressure of the baby on the bowel, low fibre and/or fluid intake, iron supplements or lack of exercise. Not only is constipation uncomfortable, but it can cause unhealthy skin and hair and block the absorption of nutrients. Calcium, zinc and magnesium deficiencies may occur in extreme cases as they are usually absorbed in the colon.

Tips to avoid or relieve constipation include:

- eat fibre-rich foods and loads of raw fruits and vegetables
- drink lots of fluids—mainly water and some fresh juices (no added sugar)
- avoid unprocessed bran—although it is very high in fibre it moves food rapidly through the body, taking essential nutrients with it
- eat small, regular meals and chew and eat food slowly
- exercise—it gets things moving
- drink warm water with a squeeze of fresh lemon juice in the morning on an empty stomach (and half an hour prior to eating) to flush out excess acids and activate the bowel
- include essential fatty acids in your diet, such as avocado, salmon or one tablespoon of flaxseed oil per day, to lubricate the bowel.

Foods to relieve constipation include:

- wholegrains, such as rye, buckwheat and wholemeal flour (and their products), wheatgerm, oats
- Dried fruit, including figs, prunes, apricots
- fresh fruit, like berries, kiwi fruit, figs, pears, lemons, banana, apples, apricots, cherries
- vegetables, such as rhubarb, avocado, peas, Brussels sprouts, potato, raw spinach, beetroot, cabbage, pumpkin, sweet potato
- fresh juices made from fresh apple, melon, prune or tomato
- legumes and dried beans (chickpeas, lentils, kidney beans)
- nuts and seeds like flaxseeds, almonds, sunflower and sesame seeds.

Haemorrhoids can also be experienced during the second and third trimesters. They are a result of strained bowel movements, relaxed muscle tone of the digestive tract, or increased blood volume. Avoiding constipation is the best form of prevention.

fLuiD ReTenTion

Bodily fluids naturally increase during pregnancy and can make you feel bloated. Ignore the urge to cut back on fluids and do exactly the opposite. You must keep drinking fluids to help flush out your system.

Salt can be a contributing factor to fluid retention and while sodium has its place in our bodily functions, we all consume enough in our diets. Sodium is present naturally in food and also hidden in processed foods. You should not need to add table salt to your meals.

Foods that help alleviate fluid retention include:

* leeks
* onions
* chives
* shallots
* green beans and celery (especially celery juice).

101

Leg cRaMPs

Leg cramps are common during the second and third trimesters, with a large percentage of expecting mums experiencing the complaint at some time during their pregnancy. Leg cramps can be an indication of a deficiency in either calcium or magnesium, with these two nutrients being the best way to overcome the discomfort. Calcium and magnesium are important nutrients in pregnancy and are nature's partners. Magnesium helps to retain calcium in the bones of both you and your baby, so it is essential to make food-rich sources a regular part of your diet.

Leg cramps in pregnancy are rarely due to a lack of salt. Food aids for leg cramps include:

* dark green, leafy vegetables—broccoli, spinach, rocket, parsley and cabbage
* nuts and seeds (pumpkin, sunflower and fennel seeds, almonds and brazil nuts)
* low-fat dairy products—skim milk powder and yoghurt
* wholegrains, including wheatgerm, buckwheat flour, brown rice and wholemeal bread

- canned fish—salmon and sardines (with bones)
- bananas (especially banana milkshakes with wheatgerm).

stretch marks

This is something that every woman, pregnant or not, seeks a remedy for. Stretch marks are the result of torn collagen bundles that occur when the skin is stressed, such as when stretching with a growing belly and breasts. But like most conditions, prevention is better than cure. Maintain healthy skin by eating foods that promote skin elasticity.

Food aids for stretch marks are:

- vitamins C and E, zinc and essential fatty acids all assist in the production of collagen—collagen keeps skin strong, supple and less inclined to tear
- protein and vitamins A, B2, B3 and B6 are all needed for healthy skin. Skin must be healthy from the inside—external creams and treatments cannot repair damage caused from within.

Other forms of prevention include:

- steady weight gain—gaining too much weight too quickly will stress the skin
- buff, exfoliate and moisturise regularly to keep skin soft and supple
- consume at least one rich source of omega 3 per day, such as a piece of grilled salmon, a tablespoon of flaxseed oil or a small handful of nuts.

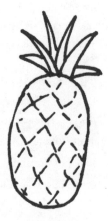

✿ recipes for second trimester
weeks 14 to 28

Poached Eggs with Spinach, Tomato and Avocado Salad

Eggs are a first-class protein and a great source of iron. Iron absorption is increased in this dish with the vitamin C-rich tomatoes and spinach. Another beneficial food combination is spinach, tomato and avocado. When these three ingredients are eaten together, the absorption of antioxidants found in each is increased. Maximum nutrition is achieved from this one very simple meal.

1 tomato

2–3 shredded basil leaves (optional)

½ cup baby spinach leaves

½ medium avocado

2 tbs white vinegar

2 eggs, preferably biodynamic

2 slices wholegrain bread, toasted

Cut the tomato in half and season with black pepper. Place under a preheated medium grill for 5 minutes, or until slightly softened. Turn off heat, sprinkle with a little of the basil leaves and leave under the grill to keep warm.

Wash, drain and finely chop the spinach leaves. Cut the avocado lengthways and thinly slice. Combine spinach, basil and avocado in a bowl. Place warmed tomatoes on top and cover. The warm tomatoes will slightly wilt the spinach and melt the avocado.

To poach the eggs, fill a deep-based frying pan or shallow saucepan with cold water and vinegar. Vinegar helps to set the egg whites. Heat the water to a very gentle simmer. Break one egg into a small, shallow bowl or large, deep spoon. Hold just above water level and carefully slide the egg into the water. Use a spoon to gently guide any stray egg white back towards the egg. Cook for 3–4 minutes for a firm yolk.

Remove the egg from the water with a slotted spoon and drain on a paper towel. Repeat with the second egg. Place one egg on each piece of toast and serve with the salad. Serves 1.

tip *To save time, try as a salad with raw tomatoes rather than grilled. Dice raw tomatoes and avocado into bite-sized pieces. Roughly chop spinach and basil and toss all ingredients into a medium bowl. Mix well to coat the leaves with the avocado and season with cracked black pepper. You could even add a splash of balsamic vinegar. Serve with poached eggs on toast.*

GOOD SOURCE OF: *protein, omega 3, folate, vitamins C, E, K and B-group, calcium, potassium, magnesium, fibre, beta-carotene, selenium*

GOOD FOR MOTHER: *immune system, sustained energy, dental problems, anaemia, skin elasticity, aiding kidney function, nourishing placenta, maximising absorption of calcium and iron, cell reproduction, protecting against cell damage*

GOOD FOR BABY: *development of brains, eyes, nervous and immune systems, hardening of bones, fuelling foetal growth*

105

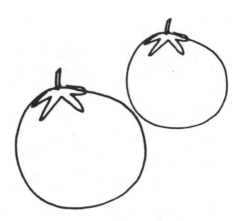

Rustic Beans and Tomatoes on Toast

This home-style 'beans on toast' is a healthy option to canned baked beans, which are often high in salt and preservatives. It can be prepared, cooked and ready to eat within 10 minutes. Protein absorption is maximised with the combination of beans and vitamin C-enriched tomatoes. You could even cook a larger batch of the beans and store in the fridge for a snack or toasted sandwich filling.

1 tbs olive oil

1 clove garlic, crushed

1 ripe tomato, diced

1 cup canned cannellini beans, thoroughly rinsed

cracked black pepper

1 tsp dried thyme or 1 tbs fresh thyme leaves

Heat oil over medium heat in a non-stick frying pan. Add garlic and gently cook for 1–2 minutes, stirring continuously.

Add tomato and cannellini beans. Cook for 2–3 minutes to heat through and soften the tomato.

Remove pan from the heat and season with pepper and herbs. Use a potato masher or back of a fork to crush the beans and tomatoes a little for a chunky consistency.

Serve with toasted soy and linseed or capeseed bread. Serves 1.

GOOD SOURCE OF: *protein, vitamins A, C, E and B-group, fibre*

GOOD FOR MOTHER: *fatigue, constipation, healthy skin, strengthening immune system, healing wounds, healthy digestive system, hypertension, converting food to fuel*

GOOD FOR BABY: *strong bone building and muscle development, eyesight, overall foetal growth*

TROPICAL C Fruit Salad

Start the day with this cleansing combination of breakfast fruits which will aid digestion and fulfil your recommended daily serving of fruit. If served with yoghurt and wholegrain toast, it makes up a complete, balanced meal. All of these fruits are incredibly rich in vitamin C, an essential nutrient throughout pregnancy and lactation. The fruits are also rich in antioxidants, which protect body cells and genetic material from any damage.

½ medium papaya and/or mango

fresh lime juice

2 kiwi fruits, peeled and sliced

½ cup blueberries

1 orange, segmented

1 passionfruit

1 cup low-fat yoghurt

107

Scoop out and discard papaya seeds and chop papaya into bite-sized pieces. Transfer to a serving bowl and cover with a good squeeze of lime juice. Set aside.

To prepare mango, slice off one cheek. Slice 3 to 4 lines across the cheek, but not through the skin and then repeat along the diagonal to form a cross-hatch pattern. Turn the skin backwards to fan out cubed mango flesh. Scoop cubes off with a spoon and place in serving bowl.

Combine all the fruit with the papaya and toss to combine. Serve with your favourite flavoured yoghurt.

GOOD SOURCE OF: *vitamins C, A, E, B2 and B12, antioxidants, fibre, calcium, protein*

GOOD FOR MOTHER: *digestion, hormone and collagen production, skin elasticity, varicose veins, healthy uterus, boosting immune system, tissue repair and healing, guarding against cell damage, normal functioning of all organs*

GOOD FOR BABY: *formation of skin and hair, eyesight, healthy placenta and body cells, strong bones, teeth and nails*

Mixed Grain Natural Muesli

There is something rewarding about making your own muesli. Don't be deterred by the lengthy list of ingredients. Most are low GI pregnancy superfoods and should be pantry staples anyway. This muesli is excellent for regular bowel function, so if constipation is proving a problem, make this a part of your daily regime. It is also rich in the B-group vitamins, which convert food to fuel. Your baby is growing rapidly now so it is imperative to provide the fuel it needs.

1 cup rolled oats

1½ cup rolled barley

½ cup rolled rye flakes

½ cup linseed, sunflower and almond meal

½ cup wheatgerm

½ cup raw pepitas

½ cup almonds or hazelnuts, roasted and roughly chopped

⅓ cup dried currants, or half-dried apricots

⅓ cup pitted prunes, roughly chopped

Combine all ingredients in an airtight container and serve portions as required with low-fat milk or yoghurt of your choice.

tip *If you prefer a crunchy, toasted muesli, spread the oats and almonds on a baking tray lined with foil. Place under a grill for 3 to 5 minutes, or until lightly browned. Cool before combining with other ingredients.*

GOOD SOURCE OF: *complex carbohydrates, B-group vitamins, calcium, zinc, magnesium, potassium, protein, fibre, essential fatty acids, antioxidants*

GOOD FOR MOTHER: *constipation, sustained energy, healthy skin, hair and eyes, digestion, metabolism, maintaining blood sugar levels, production of haemoglobin and collagen*

GOOD FOR BABY: *development of brain, spine and central nervous system, strong cell structure, bones and teeth*

Healthy Breakfast Loaf

This loaf packs a punch on flavour and nutrients. It provides most of our pregnancy needs and is a fabulous source of energy. Over-ripe bananas give a sweeter flavour but diabetics should be aware that the riper the banana, the higher its GI rating. Those at high risk of developing gestational diabetes should use bananas that have just ripened.

3 ripe bananas

1 ripe pear

1 cup plain, low-fat yoghurt

½ cup brazil nuts, chopped

2 eggs, lightly beaten

1½ cups wholemeal self-raising flour

½ cup skim milk powder

1 tsp baking powder

1 tsp nutmeg

3 tsp cinnamon

1 cup oats, or rolled barley for gluten free option

½ cup raisins

½ cup oat bran

Preheat oven to fan-forced setting of 180°C/350°F. Line a 20-cm (8-inch) loaf baking tin with baking paper.

Mash bananas into a medium-sized mixing bowl. Grate the pear into the same bowl (I like to grate over the bowl to capture all the pear juices). Add the yoghurt, nuts and lightly beaten eggs. Gently fold ingredients together.

Sift flour, skim milk powder, baking powder and spices into a large mixing bowl. Add oats, raisins and oat bran. Make a well in the centre of the dry ingredients and use a large metal spoon to gently fold through the wet ingredients.

Pour mixture into prepared baking tin. Bake for 45–50 minutes, or until the bread is cooked through. Insert a skewer to test—if cooked, the skewer will come out clean.

Allow the bread to cool in the baking tin for 10 minutes before turning out on to a wire rack to cool completely.

Slice and serve fresh, or toasted.

tip *Cut thick slices and enjoy with a fruit smoothie, or toast and spread with a little cream cheese. It is also ideal as a wholesome snack between meals. This keeps for up to three days in an airtight container stored in a dark, cool place. In the warmer months it is best kept in the fridge, where it retains its freshness for up to five days. Also suitable for freezing.*

GOOD SOURCE OF: *protein, potassium, magnesium, phosphorus, vitamins A, E and B-group including folate, selenium, fibre, calcium, essential fatty acids, complex carbohydrates*

GOOD FOR MOTHER: *fatigue, constipation, leg cramps, reproduction, skin elasticity*

GOOD FOR BABY: *fuelling foetal growth and development including skin, hair, body fat and eyesight; protecting body cells; supporting newly-functioning nervous and immune systems and blood supply*

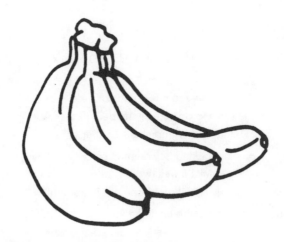

Mini Salmon Quiches

These convenient little snacks provide unquestionable nourishment and energy to support rapid foetal growth, especially brain development. The combination of salmon and egg makes this meal rich in iodine, which plays a major role in mental and physical growth.

Deficiencies can affect normal development. They will also keep you in excellent health and are the perfect portion for a snack, or can be served with a green salad and wholegrain roll as a light meal.

1 tbs olive oil

½ medium leek, thinly sliced

½ red capsicum, finely diced

3–4 shallots, finely chopped

cracked black pepper

6 eggs, preferably biodynamic

100 g (3½ oz) plain low-fat yoghurt

2 tbs finely grated parmesan cheese (optional)

1 x 210 g (7½ oz) can red salmon

1 cup baby spinach leaves, washed and roughly sliced

Preheat oven to 180°C/375°F.

Prepare muffin tin. I like to use a large (Texan) cup muffin tray for this recipe, but a regular muffin tin is fine. Individually line each muffin case with a generous square of baking paper. Mould it into the tin so that the paper forms a nice high pocket, approximately 2-cm (¾-inch) higher than the tray. This makes it easy to remove quiches from the tray without them sticking or breaking apart.

Heat the olive oil in a non-stick frying pan over medium heat. Add leek and cook for 5 minutes or until soft, stirring to prevent sticking or burning. Add capsicum and shallots and cook for a further 2–3 minutes. Remove from heat, season with cracked black pepper and set aside.

Lightly beat eggs. Whisk in yoghurt and the parmesan cheese. Add salmon, leek mixture and spinach leaves and gently fold ingredients together with a large metal spoon until combined.

Spoon mixture into muffin cases and bake for 20–25 minutes, or until browned and spongy to the touch. Remove quiches from muffin tray and serve warm with a fresh green salad, or refrigerate or freeze for later use. Makes 6 mini quiches.

tip *As your baby's brain is still maturing after birth, these quiches are beneficial during lactation. I recommend cooking and freezing them prior to the birth of your baby in preparation for those first hectic months. Quiches can be stored in an airtight container in the fridge for up to two days, or frozen for up to two months.*

GOOD SOURCE OF: *protein, omega 3, iron, zinc, iodine, calcium, folate, vitamins B12, C and D*

GOOD FOR MOTHER: *fatigue, fluid retention, bleeding gums, maintaining blood sugar levels, reflux and heartburn, hypertension, constipation, production of colostrum, anaemia*

GOOD FOR BABY: *brain and spinal development, strong bones and teeth, healthy blood*

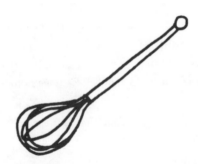

Tuna Nicoise Salad

This traditional salad has been given a protein boost. Tuna, beans and eggs are three fantastic protein sources that provide the building blocks for normal foetal growth and development. Protein is a valuable source of energy and is vital to the production of healthy blood, supporting increased blood volume and reducing the risk of developing anaemia. The enzymes in protein aid digestion and satisfy the appetite, reducing the tendency to overeat. You will feel perfectly content after this light, nourishing meal.

1 boiled egg, quartered

1 x 185 g (6½ oz) can tuna in spring water

½ punnet cherry tomatoes, halved

½ red spanish onion, thinly sliced

125 g (4 oz) canned cannellini beans,
   rinsed thoroughly

100 g (3½ oz) green beans, cut into bite-sized lengths

⅓ cup fresh parsley and chives/parsley and basil

dressing:

2 tbs extra virgin olive oil

1 tbs lemon juice

1 tsp Dijon mustard

salt and pepper

113

Fill a small saucepan with cold water and add the egg. Slowly bring the water to a steady simmer and cook for 5–7 minutes.

Prepare the dressing by combining all ingredients in a jar and whisk or shake vigorously.

Place tuna into a large salad bowl and pour half of the dressing over to flavour the tuna. Set aside.

Prepare vegetables and cannellini beans. Add these to the tuna, with the exception of the green beans.

Remove cooked eggs from the saucepan. Do not discard the water. Rinse the eggs under cold water. This will stop the cooking process and make the eggs easier to handle.

Using the same saucepan and water, steam the beans for 1–2 minutes. Add to salad.

Peel the eggs and cut into quarters. Add to the salad, together with the chopped herbs.

Mix ingredients together and dress with remaining dressing. Season with cracked black pepper.

GOOD SOURCE OF: *protein, iodine, zinc, folate, omega 3, calcium, potassium, vitamins A, C, D and B-group*

GOOD FOR MOTHER: *digestion, fluid retention, anaemia, bleeding gums, skin elasticity, increased blood supply, nourishing placenta, complete calcium function, reducing risk of osteoporosis*

GOOD FOR BABY: *rapid foetal growth, development of brain, nervous and immune systems, formation of muscles, skin, hair and body fat, hardening of bones*

Lentil and Almond Salad

This dish is ideal for vegetarians as lentils and nuts combine to provide all of the essential amino acids. It also has a low GI rating so is suitable for diabetics or those at high risk of developing gestational diabetes. Not only that, this recipe is fantastic for constipation and an excellent source of energy for both mother and growing baby. It is a substantial meal on its own, or is delicious with cooked and shredded chicken breast stirred through.

½ cup dried brown lentils/1 x 400 g (14 oz) canned lentils

½ tsp fennel seeds, lightly pan-roasted and ground

½ cup almonds, roughly chopped

1 small red capsicum, finely diced

⅓ cup currants

½ red onion, finely diced

½ cup finely sliced green beans/diced fennel bulb

½ cup fresh parsley or spinach, chopped

cracked black pepper

1–2 tbs flaxseed oil

115

Rinse lentils through a strainer. Place in a medium saucepan with 4 cups of water. Bring to the boil and cook for 10–15 minutes, or until al dente. Be careful not to overcook as lentils will turn mushy. Alternatively, drain and thoroughly rinse canned lentils.

Heat a frying pan over a medium heat. Dry fry fennel seeds and almonds for a few minutes, or until seeds become aromatic, being careful not to burn. Transfer from pan into a mortar and pestle. Gently bash to release the flavour of the fennel seeds and to crush the almonds. If you do not have a mortar and pestle, roughly chop on a chopping board.

Prepare all other ingredients, except the flaxseed oil and black pepper, and place into a large serving bowl with almonds and fennel seeds.

Strain and rinse lentils. Shake off all excess water and add lentils to salad mixture. Season with black pepper and drizzle over the flaxseed oil. Toss to combine.

Serve with a dollop of yoghurt or cooked, shredded chicken breast.

GOOD SOURCE OF: *protein, fibre, calcium, iron, magnesium, potassium, phosphorus, vitamins A, C, E, K and B-group, including folate, essential fatty acids*

GOOD FOR MOTHER: *vegetarians, constipation, gestational diabetes, fatigue, digestion, circulation, hypertension, skin elasticity, production of red blood cells, normal blood clotting, toning uterus, immunity, cell growth, maintaining healthy organs, blood, skin, teeth and nails, strong bones*

GOOD FOR BABY: *development of brain and central nervous system*

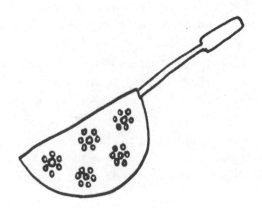

Beetroot, pumpkin and spinach salad

This recipe is excellent for healthy blood, skin and eyes. Beetroot is fantastic for the liver and the blood and so this salad is ideally suited to the second trimester when your body is producing extra blood to maintain your pregnancy. It will also reduce the risk of developing anaemia. Serve with grilled meat or chicken, or add a cup of chickpeas for a complete protein meal source for vegetarians.

1 large or 2 medium beetroots	*dressing*:
½ pumpkin	2 tbs fresh orange juice
⅓ cup walnuts	1 tbs grapeseed or extra virgin olive oil
100 g (3½ oz) green beans/1 bunch	1 tsp wholegrain mustard
fresh asparagus	1 small garlic clove, crushed
1½ cups English spinach leaves,	cracked black pepper
finely shredded	
1 cup cooked chickpeas (complete protein option)	

117

Preheat oven to 200°C/400°F. Wrap beetroot in foil and roast for 40 minutes.

Cut pumpkin into 4-cm or bite-sized pieces and place on a baking tray lined with baking paper. I like to leave the skin on my pumpkin as it is delicious when roasted, but this is a personal choice. Wash the skin thoroughly if you do choose to eat it. Place the pumpkin into the oven with the beetroot and roast for 30 minutes.

Spread walnuts on to a flat baking tray and pop into the oven. Roast for 4–5 minutes, being careful not to burn them.

Place all dressing ingredients into a jar and shake vigorously.

Once the beetroot is cooked, unwrap the foil and push the skin off. It should slide off very easily; if not, the beetroot may not be properly cooked. (You may wish to wear surgical gloves as your hands will take on the colour of the beetroot, but this does come off easily with soap and water.)

Remove the top stem and thin roots of the beetroot and while still warm cut into segments. Place beetroot in a bowl and pour over half the dressing. Set aside to marinate while you prepare the salad.

Wash and trim the beans. Cut into 3 cm lengths and steam for 1–2 minutes.

Place the beans, walnuts, spinach and pumpkin into a large salad bowl. Pour the beetroot and its juices into the salad, together with the remaining dressing. Toss to combine and serve warm.

GOOD SOURCE OF: *vitamins A, C, E, K and B-group including folate, potassium, magnesium, protein, calcium, zinc, fibre*

GOOD FOR MOTHER: *anaemia, increased blood supply, healthy liver and kidneys, immunity, constipation, hypertension, fertility, dental problems, vegetarians*

GOOD FOR BABY: *healthy cell growth, strong bones, healthy skin and eyes, development of brain and nervous system, formation of muscles, skin, hair and body fat, nourishing placenta*

118

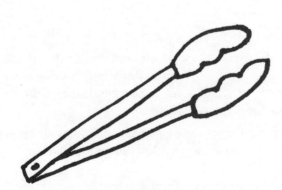

Aunt Jill's Carrot and Ginger Soup

This is a delicious alternative to pumpkin soup. Carrots have a much lower GI rating than their orange cousins, and the soup is rich in antioxidants to help build resistance to infections, colds and flu. They also protect cells and genetic material.

1 tbs olive oil

2 brown onions, diced

1 clove garlic, crushed

6 medium-sized carrots, roughly sliced into bite-sized pieces

2 sticks celery, diced

1 green capsicum, diced

2 tsp fresh ginger, finely grated

3 cups (750 ml/24 fl oz) chicken stock

cracked black pepper

2–3 tsp fresh coriander, finely chopped

Heat oil over a medium heat in a large cooking pot. Gently cook onion and garlic for about 5 minutes, or until soft. Add carrots, celery, capsicum, ginger and chicken stock. Bring to the boil, then reduce to a simmer. Cover the pot and cook for 30 minutes, or until carrots have softened. Transfer soup mixture into a food processor and blend to a smooth puree. Season with black pepper and the fresh coriander. Serve with a dollop of plain yoghurt.

 For a creamy version of this soup, add 1 cup of low-fat evaporated milk.

GOOD SOURCE OF: *beta-carotene, antioxidants, dietary fibre, vitamin C, protein, potassium, antioxidants*

GOOD FOR MOTHER: *reflux and heartburn, nausea, food aversions, constipation, diabetes, digestion, relieving flatulence, fluid retention, skin elasticity, circulation*

GOOD FOR BABY: *strong immune system, healthy skin, hair and nails, eyesight, reproduction of cells*

Chickpea, Rosemary and Tomato Soup

Chickpeas are a wonder food. They are very economical, low in saturated fat, high in protein and when eaten with grains they are a complete non-animal protein source. Ideally, serve this soup with mixed grain bread, such as soy and linseed. Alternatively, add ½ cup of cooked risone pasta to the soup when you add the chickpeas and stock to the recipe. This will yield a thicker, heartier soup.

400 g (14 oz) cooked chickpeas or 170 g (5½ oz) dried chickpeas

2 tbs olive oil

1 large brown onion or leek (white part only)

8 sprigs rosemary, leaves removed and finely chopped from 4 of the sprigs

4 cloves garlic, crushed

2 x 400 g (14 oz) can diced tomatoes, salt reduced

2½ cups (600 ml/20 fl oz) chicken stock

If using dried chickpeas, soak and cook according to packet directions. If using canned chickpeas, drain and rinse thoroughly.

Heat oil over low-medium heat in a large cooking pot. Saute leek/onion for 3 minutes, until soft and golden. Add chopped rosemary, rosemary sprigs and garlic and continue cooking for 2–3 minutes. Add tomatoes, together with ½ cup of the stock. Reduce to a simmer, cover and cook for 20 minutes.

Puree half of the chickpeas with ½ cup of the stock. Add chickpea puree to the tomato mixture along with the whole chickpeas and remaining 1½ cups stock. Cover and simmer for a further 20 minutes. Remove whole rosemary sprigs prior to serving.

tip *Store in the refrigerator for up to 3 days. Also suitable for freezing.*

GOOD SOURCE OF: *protein, iron, calcium, vitamins A, C and B-group, fibre, potassium, magnesium*

GOOD FOR MOTHER: *fatigue, anaemia, heartburn, reflux, food aversions, hypertension, constipation, healthy blood, skin and eyes*

GOOD FOR BABY: *overall foetal growth, development of major organs and circulatory systems*

Steak sandwich with Tomato salsa

This is one of the best meals to nourish your blood. Tomatoes and spinach/rocket are rich in vitamin C to enhance iron absorption from the steak. When steak is eaten with hummus, dark salad leaves and wholegrain bread, the amount of folate absorbed is increased. And the olive oil in the salsa brings out additional antioxidant properties in the tomatoes. All of these nutrients assist in healthy red blood cell production to support the extra blood volume of you and your baby. Add to this the marvels of beetroot in oxygenating the blood and aiding liver function, and you will have very minimal chance of developing anaemia. The hummus, dark leaves and wholegrain bread are also great sources of calcium for strong teeth and bones.

2 x 100 g (3½ oz) lean steaks

handful of rocket or spinach leaves

2–3 slices cooked beetroot

4 thick slices wholemeal bread

hummus, to serve

tomato salsa:

2 tomatoes, diced

½ red onion, diced

2 tbs fresh basil leaves

1 tsp olive oil

1 small clove garlic (optional)

small pinch iodised salt

Preheat grill or barbeque. Trim steak of visible fat and baste with a little olive oil.

Prepare tomato salsa by combining all ingredients in a medium bowl. Mix well and set aside at room temperature.

Place steak on grill or barbeque and cook to your liking. Meanwhile, wash and pat dry salad leaves, prepare beetroot and lightly toast the bread. Spread the toast with hummus. Scoop the salsa on two slices of toast. Follow this with the steak, beetroot and salad leaves and top with remaining slices of toast. Cut in half and serve.

GOOD SOURCE OF: *iron, protein, vitamins C and B-group especially B12, calcium, magnesium, fibre, antioxidants, essential fatty acids*

GOOD FOR MOTHER: *healthy blood, anaemia, fatigue, iron absorption, nourishing all major organs of both mother and baby*

GOOD FOR BABY: *strong healthy teeth and bones, growth of muscles, skin, hair, body fat*

Leek and Mushroom frittata

This dish provides *all* of your nutritional needs for pregnancy. Eggs are close to being a complete food source and they create the base of this frittata. Calcium requirements double during pregnancy and this dish certainly fulfils those needs. It is also rich in vitamin D and magnesium to complete the proper function of calcium. This meal promotes strong, healthy teeth and bones and reduces the risk of osteoporosis later in life. Can be served for brunch, lunch or dinner.

1 tbs olive oil

1 leek, white part only, thinly sliced

2 cloves garlic, crushed

400 g (14 oz) button mushrooms, sliced

1 cup English spinach, roughly shredded

8 eggs

½ cup plain low-fat yoghurt

⅓ cup parmesan or tasty cheese

Preheat oven to 180°C/350°F. Line a 24-cm (9½-inch) round quiche dish or cake tin with baking paper.

Heat oil in a non-stick frying pan over a medium–low heat. Add leek and cook for 3–4 minutes until soft, being careful not to burn or over-brown. Add garlic and mushrooms and cook for another 3 minutes, stirring continuously. Turn heat off and stir through the spinach leaves. Set aside.

Lightly beat the eggs in a large mixing bowl. Add yoghurt and cheese and beat on a low speed for 1 minute. Use a large, metal spoon and gently fold leek mixture through the eggs.

Pour mixture into the prepared pan and bake for 20 minutes, or until eggs are set and golden brown. Rest the frittata for 5 minutes before turning on to a plate for serving. Delicious warm or cold, served with a mixed leaf and tomato salad. Serves 6–8 and keeps for up to 3–4 days in the refrigerator.

Asparagus, red capsicum and chives are also great ingredients for frittatas.

GOOD SOURCE OF: *iodine, zinc, omega 3, vitamins A, C, D, K, B6 and B12, folate, calcium, protein, phosphorus, potassium, magnesium, selenium*

GOOD FOR MOTHER: *fatigue, digestion, fluid retention, leg cramps, healthy kidneys, dental problems, reducing risk of osteoporosis, lactation, nourishing placenta*

GOOD FOR BABY: *brain and physical development, strong healthy bones, teeth and nails, production of red blood cells, eyesight, growth of skin, muscles, hair, fat cells and major organs*

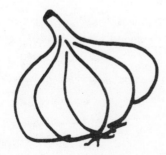

GriLLeD VegeTable SKeweRs with Hummus

This recipe is rich in calcium and the chickpeas and sesame seeds in hummus makes it a complete protein source for vegetarians. Mushrooms are another invaluable source of nutrition as they promote red blood cell production, reducing the risk of anaemia.

12 medium-sized mushrooms

12 cherry tomatoes

2 zucchini, cut into 2-cm (¾-inch) cubes

6 skewers

hummus to serve (see page 203)

marinade:

1 tbs extra virgin olive oil

3 tsp balsamic vinegar

1 tbs fresh basil or parsley, finely chopped

cracked black pepper

If using wooden skewers, soak in water for 30 minutes to prevent burning.

Combine marinade ingredients in a medium bowl. Prepare vegetables and marinate for 15–20 minutes, longer if time allows. Thread vegetables on to skewer in the following order: zucchini, mushroom, tomato; zucchini, mushroom tomato; zucchini. Repeat with remaining skewers.

Preheat oven grill to a medium heat. Place skewers under the grill and cook for 8–10 minutes, turning regularly to brown evenly. Skewers can also be cooked over a low heat on the barbeque.

Serve skewers with the hummus. This dish can be served with brown rice or in a wholegrain roll. It is also a wonderful side to any grilled meat.

GOOD SOURCE OF: *protein, calcium, iron, vitamins D, B6 and B12, folate, fibre, magnesium, potassium, phosphorus*

GOOD FOR MOTHER: *vegetarians, fatigue, constipation, diabetes, digestion, skin elasticity, healthy blood and kidneys, reducing risk of osteoporosis, anaemia and dental problems*

GOOD FOR BABY: *growth of muscles, skin and hair, hardening of bones and external structure*

seafood stew

This is probably one of the easiest, tastiest and nourishing recipes in this book. In fact, I would highly recommend you continue eating this dish through to lactation. It provides close to all of the nutrients essential to a healthy pregnancy and is particularly rich in zinc and iodine. It is very easy to become deficient in these two nutrients as their sources are fairly limited, and yet they are absolutely vital to normal and proper development of the brain and central nervous system. The stew is also rich in omega 3 and protein. Put simply, this dish is brain food for both you and your baby.

1 tbs olive oil

1 leek or large brown onion

3 garlic cloves, crushed

½ tsp sweet paprika

1 x 400 g (14 oz) canned diced tomatoes

½ cup water

2 bay leaves

2 tsp dried thyme

10 fresh mussels, in their shells

1 snapper fillet

1 salmon fillet

100 g (3½ oz) calamari rings

½ cup fresh parsley, chopped

125

Finely slice the leek/onion and prepare the garlic.

Heat the olive oil in a heavy-based frying pan with a lid. Cook the leeks/onion for 4–5 minutes, or until soft. Add garlic and cook for a further 2 minutes before adding the paprika and continue cooking for another minute or two. Add tomatoes, water, bay leaf and thyme. Season generously with black pepper. Bring sauce to a gentle simmer, cover and cook for 10 minutes.

Meanwhile, prepare the seafood. Place mussels in a colander and rinse under cold, running water. Scrub the mussel shells to remove any barnacles and pull out the 'hairy beards'. Give them a final rinse with cold water and leave to drain.

Cut the fish fillets into 3 cm pieces, removing the skin. Combine with the calamari rings.

Once the tomato mixture has cooked for 10 minutes, add the seafood. Gently stir through and coat with the sauce. Cover the pan and cook for 3–4 minutes shaking the pan once or twice.

Check to see fish is cooked through. Remove the bay leaves and any mussels that have not opened. Dislodge the mussels from their shells. Discard shells and add the mussels to the stew.

Stir through fresh parsley and serve with any of the above-mentioned carbohydrate accompaniments. A small bowl of steamed greens is also recommended. Serve with warm, crusty wholegrain bread to soak up the broth.

 This meal can be ready to serve within 30 minutes. It is extremely versatile, too. Add pasta for a delicious marinara dish, or stir through some rice for a thicker, heartier stew.

Canned tomatoes are one of the rare cases where little nutritional value is lost during the canning process. They are the perfect pantry staple for quick-and-easy meals. Always read the labels and choose salt-reduced and no-added sugar brands.

GOOD SOURCE OF: *zinc, iodine, omega 3, iron, protein, calcium, potassium, phosphorus, selenium, vitamins A, C, D, E and B-group, antioxidants*

GOOD FOR MOTHER: *fertility, reducing risk of pre-term birth, increased blood volume, energy source, immunity, iron and calcium absorption, nourishing placenta and uterus, anaemia, dental problems, hypertension, skin elasticity*

GOOD FOR BABY: *development of baby's brain, immune and central nervous systems, supporting growth of cells, muscles, skin, hair and body fat, eyesight, hard structure of teeth, bones and all cells*

snapper with summer salsa

If you could serve summertime on a plate—bursting with goodness from the ocean, bright, fresh, colourful and carefree—this would be it. It can be made, on the table and ready to eat in under 20 minutes, so there's no fuss and absolutely no excuse to not try this recipe. It is a very light meal and is perfect for the second trimester.

2 snapper fillets

2 tsp olive oil

salsa:

2 nectarines or peaches, washed and diced

½ red capsicum, finely diced

½ avocado, finely diced

2 shallots, finely diced

8 fresh mint leaves, finely shredded

juice of 1 lime

150 g (5 oz) green beans, steamed to serve

127

Prepare the salsa by combining the nectarines, capsicum, avocado, shallots and mint. Squeeze over lime juice and stir through. Set aside at room temperature to allow flavours to develop.

Use a sharp knife and cut 2–3 slashes into the skin of the fish. This will prevent the fish from curling up during cooking. Baste each fillet with 1 teaspoon of olive oil and season with black pepper.

Heat a non-stick frying pan and cook fillets for 3 minutes on each side, or until cooked through. Fish is cooked when the flesh turns opaque and flakes easily with a fork. Remove the fish from the pan immediately as the fish will continue cooking for a minute or so once removed from the heat. If your fish tastes a little rubbery, you have overcooked the fillet.

Pile a generous amount of salsa on top of each fish fillet and serve with the steamed greens. Baked sweet potato wedges or a small bowl of rice are good accompaniments to this dish.

tip *This summer salsa also complements chicken and pork.*

GOOD SOURCE OF: *omega 3, protein, iron, iodine, zinc, potassium, vitamins A, C, D, K and B-group*

GOOD FOR MOTHER: *digestion, circulation, stretch marks, toning and nourishing the uterus, immunity, lactation, dental problems, healthy skin, hair and eyes for both mother and baby*

GOOD FOR BABY: *production of body cells, brain development, strong bones, brain/ nerve impulses, formation of body fat, eyesight, physical growth, including muscles and skin*

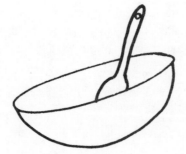

Teriyaki Salmon with Broccolini and Brown Rice

This would have to be the easiest main course in this book. Salmon is pure brain food, but it is also rich in many other essential nutrients that promote physical growth and development of your unborn. The broccolini and rice serve to complement the goodness of the fish. Teriyaki sauce is available in most supermarkets and goes exceptionally well with the salmon.

> 2 x 150 g (5 oz) salmon fillets
>
> 2 tbs teriyaki sauce
>
> ½ cup uncooked brown rice
>
> 1 bunch broccolini or broccoli

Pour the teriyaki sauce over the salmon fillets. Cover with plastic wrap and marinate in the refrigerator for 15–30 minutes, or longer if time permits.

Cook rice according to packet directions. Wash and trim vegetables and prepare a steamer for cooking.

Preheat the oven grill to a medium heat. A high heat will burn the marinade.

Place the salmon fillets skin-side down on a grill tray. Cook under the grill for 8–10 minutes, depending on the thickness of the fillet. While the fish is cooking, steam the vegetables for about 4 minutes.

Serve the salmon with brown rice and vegetables.

129

GOOD SOURCE OF: *zinc, iodine, omega 3, protein, iron, vitamin B12, folate, fibre*

GOOD FOR MOTHER: *skin elasticity, fertility, lactation, growing placenta, immunity, healthy heart, hypertension, constipation, anaemia*

GOOD FOR BABY: *brain and spinal development, strong bone and cell structure, healthy blood supply, development of major organs, foetal growth, including skin, hair and body fat, eyesight*

SPiceD CRusteD SaLmon with white Bean PuRee

This dish should assist with any digestion problems you may experience. The spices used to crust the salmon are all known to assist digestion and some are also useful for nausea. You may have been told to avoid spicy foods if suffering from heartburn and reflux, but it is usually the more hot spices such as chilli that cause complaint.

½ tsp whole fennel seeds

1 tsp coriander

1 tsp cumin

½ tsp paprika

½ tsp sea salt

cracked black pepper

2 x 150 g (5 oz) salmon fillet

200 g broccoli and green beans to serve

white bean puree:

1 x 400 g (14 oz) canned cannelloni beans

1 tbs lemon juice

½ small clove garlic, crushed

2 tbs olive oil

cracked black pepper

Preheat oven to 180°C/350°F and prepare a baking tray to cook the fish.

Grind fennel seeds in a mortar and pestle or spice grinder. Add other spices and a few twists of black pepper. Thoroughly combine the spices and pour on to a plate or flat surface. Press the skinless side of the salmon into the spices and use your fingers to press it firmly into the fillets. If time allows, stand for 15–30 minutes to flavour the fish.

To make the white bean puree, drain and thoroughly rinse beans under cold water. Place beans, lemon juice and garlic into a food processor and blend until combined. With the processor still running, slowly add the olive oil. Blend to form a smooth puree. If the mixture seems a little dry or lumpy add a little more olive oil to form a creamy consistency. Alternatively, place all ingredients into a bowl and puree with hand blender. Season to taste with black pepper.

Prepare vegetables for light steaming while you cook the fish.

Heat 1 tablespoon olive oil in a non-stick frying pan over a medium heat. Add salmon fillets, spice-side down, and cook for 2–3 minutes or until spices are lightly browned.

Transfer to baking tray and bake for 5–8 minutes, or until the fillet is cooked through. You will be able to determine this by checking the sides of the salmon where you can see the flesh turning opaque as it cooks in towards the centre. Timing will depend on the thickness of the fillet.

Serve salmon on a bed of white bean puree, together with the steamed beans and broccoli.

 It is important to thoroughly combine spices to deliver an evenly distributed flavour. I find shaking the mixture in a glass jar or airtight container is most effective. The longer spice mixes are allowed to stand, the more the flavours amalgamate. If this is a favourite recipe, double or even triple the spice quantities and store in an airtight jar in a dark, cool place. Flavours will improve with age.

For a different take on this spice mix, combine 1 tbs of spice mix with 1 clove of crushed garlic, 1 tbs lemon juice and ¼ cup yoghurt. Marinate salmon in the spiced yoghurt for 15 minutes and bake in a moderate oven for 15–20 minutes. Delicious.

Cook one or two extra spiced salmon fillets—they are fabulous flaked through a salad of rocket leaves, shallots and diced tomatoes.

Serve spiced salmon with yoghurt as a substitute to the white bean puree.

131

GOOD SOURCE OF: *omega 3, iodine, zinc, protein, iron, calcium, fibre, vitamins C and B-group*

GOOD FOR MOTHER: *digestion, constipation, production of reproductive hormones, skin elasticity, nourishing placenta, boosting immunity, normal blood clotting, healthy heart and blood, hypertension, diabetes, constipation*

GOOD FOR BABY: *brain development and brain function, eyesight, strong bone and cell structure, fantastic fuel source, formation of all major organs*

Red Capsicums Stuffed with Sardines

I must admit, I was never partial to sardines. In fact I strongly disliked them, but after discovering their amazing nutritional value—they are extremely rich in calcium and omega 3—I had to find a way to disguise their strong flavour and include them in my diet. This is now one of my favourite meals and is a delicious way to reap the unbeatable goodness of this little fish. The recipe has a very low GI rating for sustained energy.

½ cup basmati rice

1 tbs olive oil

2 cloves garlic, crushed

185 g (6½ oz) can sardines in spring water, drained

juice and zest of one lemon

1 tbs currants

½ cup pine nuts

½ cup fresh parsley, finely chopped

cracked black pepper

1 red capsicum, deseeded and cut in half horizontally

2 tbs wheatgerm

Preheat oven to 180°C/350°F. Line a baking tray with baking paper.

Cook rice according to packet directions.

Meanwhile, heat olive oil in a non-stick frying pan over medium heat. Gently cook garlic for 1–2 minutes. Add sardines, lemon zest, currants, pine nuts and a squeeze of lemon juice to moisten the mixture. Cook for 1 minute before removing from heat.

Drain and rinse rice. Add rice and parsley to the sardine mixture. Season with cracked black pepper and combine. Spoon into red capsicum cases and generously sprinkle wheatgerm over the top. Bake for 25 minutes and serve with a salad of your choice. Serves 1.

For an extra boost of calcium, add two tablespoons of grated cheddar cheese. Chopped spinach is also a great nutritional addition.

GOOD SOURCE OF: *calcium, omega 3, essential fatty acids, zinc, iodine, folate, beta-carotene, vitamins C and B-group, antioxidants, magnesium*

GOOD FOR MOTHER: *dental problems, anaemia, constipation, diabetes, hypertension, fatigue, stretch marks, nourishing uterus, healthy kidneys, blood supply, lactation, reducing risk of osteoporosis, normal blood clotting*

GOOD FOR BABY: *bones hardening, rapid organ growth, including brain, muscles, lungs, skin, hair and body fat, development of immune and nervous systems, muscle contractions and nerve function*

133

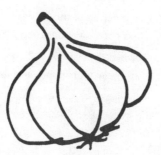

Chicken and Soba Noodle Salad

This salad is bursting with all the goodies needed for pregnancy. It is light and refreshing and would also suit the third trimester, when smaller meals are called for. Soba noodles are available in the Asian foods section of most supermarkets. They are made from buckwheat, which is a wholegrain and a fabulous nutritional food source. It helps to strengthen and tone the walls of blood capillaries to help reduce the onset of varicose veins. Buckwheat also aids digestion and promotes the absorption of nutrients by the body so you can enjoy this dish knowing that every single mouthful counts.

135 g (4½ oz) organic soba noodles

½ bunch baby bok choy

1 medium head broccoli

10 snow peas

2 tbs pepitas

2 tbs sesame seeds

½ cup fresh coriander, chopped

2 cooked chicken breasts, shredded

dressing:

4 tbs fresh lime juice

2 tbs rice wine vinegar

½–1 tsp fresh red chilli, chopped

2 tbs honey

2 tbs grape seed oil

Cook soba noodles according to packet directions. I like to break the noodles into short lengths prior to cooking, which makes them easier to both prepare and eat. Once cooked, rinse noodles immediately under cold water and separate with your hands to prevent them from clumping. Place in a colander to drain.

Cut the base off the bok choy and separate the leaves. Wash and dry thoroughly. Cut broccoli into small florets and cut snow peas diagonally in half.

Toast pepitas and sesame seeds in a dry pan for 2–3 minutes, or until just golden brown. Shake the pan regularly to prevent burning and remove from pan as soon as they are toasted.

Lightly steam the bok choy and broccoli for 2–3 minutes. Add the snow peas and steam for the final minute only.

Mix all ingredients together in a bowl with the soba noodles. Drizzle with the dressing and toss to coat the salad.

tip *This salad is the perfect picnic partner or work lunch. It can be pre-made up to the point of dressing the salad. Cover the prepared salad in plastic wrap or store in an airtight container and keep chilled until needed. Add the dressing just prior to serving.*

GOOD SOURCE OF: *vitamins A, C, E and B-group especially folate, calcium, protein, iron, fibre, antioxidants, potassium, essential fatty acids*

GOOD FOR MOTHER: *gluten-free diet, diabetes, fatigue, dental problems, iron absorption, healthy blood, normal liver and kidney function, stretch marks, circulation, strengthening blood capillaries*

GOOD FOR BABY: *development of neural tube, brain and nervous system, production of increased blood supply, promoting cell growth and protecting against damage, strong bone structure, boosting immune system, healthy skin, teeth and gums*

135

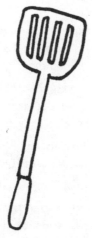

Chicken and Thai Basil Stir-fry

If your stir-fries aren't already creating a sensation, it may be that you haven't yet discovered Thai basil. It is the secret ingredient to creating that authentic Thai flavour and this delicious classic dish uses a full cup of this wonderfully fragrant herb. Stir-fries are a very healthy and tasty way to eat loads of vegetables, herbs and spices. Cooking time is only 5–10 minutes, which minimises the amount of nutrients lost during cooking.

4 cloves garlic, crushed

3 cm piece peeled fresh ginger

½ long red chilli

400 g (14 oz) chicken breast fillets

½ red capsicum, thinly sliced

½ bunch garlic shoots, cut into 3-cm (1¼-inch) lengths

1 bunch asparagus, cut into 3-cm (1¼-inch) lengths (or 100 g/3½ oz broccoli)

2 shallots, sliced diagonally

1 cup Thai basil leaves, left whole

2 tbs chicken stock (salt reduced or homemade)

2 tbs oyster sauce

1 tbs grapeseed or canola oil

136

Use the fine side of a grater and grate the garlic and ginger. Finely slice the chilli and place these three ingredients into a mortar and pestle and pound to form a paste. This can also be done in a food processor.

Trim chicken breast of visible fat. Rinse under cold water and pat dry with paper towel. Finely slice the chicken along the grain of the meat. Place chicken in a bowl and add the chilli paste. Thoroughly coat the chicken with the paste and set aside.

Wash and prepare all vegetables and place into a bowl, with the exception of the shallots and Thai basil. Place those in a separate bowl to be added at the end of cooking.

Measure out stock and oyster sauce and mix together.

Heat the oil in a hot wok. Add the chicken and paste and stir-fry for 1–2 minutes or until chicken is seared on all sides. Add the garlic shoots, red capsicum and asparagus. Cook for a further minute before adding the stock and sauce. Continue stir-frying, tossing and coating all ingredients with the sauce. Do this for 2 minutes and finally add the Thai basil and shallots. Cook for another 30 seconds, or until the basil leaves have just wilted.

Serve with steamed rice if desired.

 The secret to a successful stir-fry is to work quickly. To do this you must have all ingredients prepared and ready to go. This includes measuring out sauces, stock and other liquids. Cutting ingredients to a similar length and thickness is another useful tip, and the smaller the better. The vegetables will then cook evenly in less time. Combine those ingredients that will be added to the stir-fry at the same time, enabling you to work efficiently. Fresh herbs should always be added just prior to serving. Toss them through the dish and continue cooking for 30 seconds to flavour. Thai basil and garlic shoots can be found in all Asian grocery stores and the larger supermarkets.

137

GOOD SOURCE OF: *protein, iron, phosphorus, potassium, selenium, beta-carotene, vitamins C, K, B6 and B12, folate, fibre*

GOOD FOR MOTHER: *anaemia, red blood cell production, fatigue, circulation, toning heart muscles, hypertension, digestion, immunity (particularly good for cold and flus), iron absorption*

GOOD FOR BABY: *rapid foetal growth, development of central nervous system, eyesight, healthy bones, teeth and skin, cell growth*

chicken and corn wraps

This is my healthy version of the Mexican tortilla and can be prepared within 30 minutes. It is light, refreshing and highly nutritious. Corn belongs to the wholegrain food group and is a great source of dietary fibre and B vitamins. By combining the iron source, chicken, with the salsa, which is rich in vitamin C, you increase your ability to ward off anaemia, most common in the second trimester.

250 g (9 oz) chicken breast fillets

1 serving of corn salsa (see recipe page 231)

4 corn mountain bread wraps

Trim fat from chicken breasts and slice in half lengthwise for two evenly sized fillets. Place fillets in a saucepan of simmering water. Gently poach chicken for 5 minutes, or until cooked through.

Remove chicken from the saucepan and place on a plate lined with baking paper to absorb any excess liquid. Shred or finely slice the chicken and stir through the corn salsa.

Arrange four sheets of mountain bread on a clean, flat surface. Divide the chicken and salsa evenly between the four sheets. Place the mixture at one end of each sheet, about 2-cm (¾-inch) from the side edges to prevent mixture from falling out during cooking and eating. Tuck side edges in and roll up into a secure wrap.

Heat a medium-sized, shallow frying pan. Place the wraps into the dry pan and lightly brown on each side. Squeeze some fresh lime juice over the top and serve warm.

GOOD SOURCE OF: *protein, iron, phosphorus, potassium, magnesium, selenium, zinc, vitamins A, C, E, K and B-group, omega 3, complex carbohydrates, fibre*

GOOD FOR MOTHER: *hypertension, fluid retention, skin elasticity, healthy skin, hair, eyes and blood, constipation, energy source, fatigue, immunity, anaemia, nourishing placenta, normal blood clotting, iron absorption, dental problems, leg cramps*

GOOD FOR BABY: *supporting rapid foetal growth including muscles, skin, hair and body fat, development of brain, nervous and immune systems, strong cell structure, eyesight*

BBQ Lamb with Barley, Artichoke and Asparagus Salad

Please try this recipe. The ingredients might seem a little out of the ordinary, but the combination is sensational in both flavour and nutrition. Every single ingredient is a superfood for pregnancy, so I don't even need to express how good this simple meal is for you and your growing baby.

Barley is a fabulous alternative to rice or pasta. It has more nutritional value and is just as easy to prepare. It is available from supermarkets and often called pearl barley. Its low GI rating makes it ideal for diabetes and it's also suited to a gluten-free diet.

Artichokes are fantastic for the health of your liver, which is working overtime to cleanse and filter your increased blood supply. In fact, this is a very cleansing dish, with most of the ingredients working to detoxify the body of impurities. Great for the health of the heart, kidneys and blood supply.

This barley salad serves as a complete protein source beneficial to vegetarians and is a great work lunch. Prepare all ingredients with the exception of parsley, which should always be chopped just prior to serving.

139

½ cup uncooked barley (to yield 1½ cups cooked)

400 g (16 oz) lamb fillets

olive oil

100 g (3½ oz) marinated artichokes (in jar, not open deli counter)

1 bunch asparagus or green beans

½ cup grated parmesan cheese

½ cup parsley, finely chopped

dressing:

1 tbs fresh lemon juice

2 tsp flaxseed oil

cracked black pepper

Thoroughly rinse barley and place in a saucepan with 3 cups of water. Gently boil for 25–30 minutes, or until al dente.

Preheat a barbeque or grill to a medium-high heat. Trim lamb fillets of any visible fat and lightly baste with olive oil.

While barley is cooking, drain the artichokes and slice into quarters and lightly steam asparagus. Place ingredients into a medium salad bowl with the cheese and parsley.

Combine flaxseed oil, lemon juice and lots of black pepper in a jar or small cup. Whisk vigorously to combine. Set aside.

Towards the end of the barley cooking time, cook the lamb fillets. They will need approximately 4–5 minutes on each side, depending on the thickness of the fillet. Once cooked, transfer to a warm plate and cover with foil. Rest the meat for 5 minutes prior to slicing.

Strain the barley and rinse with warm water. Add it to the salad bowl, along with the dressing, and mix ingredients together. Divide and arrange the salad in the centre of each serving plate. Slice the lamb diagonally into 2 cm thick slices and arrange on top of the barley salad. Season with extra cracked black pepper as desired.

 This dish is also fabulous drizzled with pumpkin oil. Pumpkin oil can be found in all health food shops and is a highly nutritious source of omega 6 and omega 9. The barley salad is also a perfect accompaniment to grilled white fish.

GOOD SOURCE OF: *protein, iron, calcium, potassium, phosphorus, magnesium, fibre, vitamins A, C, K and B-group, especially folate and B12*

GOOD FOR MOTHER: *liver function, fatigue, anaemia, digestive system, circulation, constipation, hypertension, leg cramps, healthy skin, strong capillary walls, production of healthy red blood cells, absorption of iron and calcium, nourishing placenta, gluten free diets*

GOOD FOR BABY: *development of brain, nervous and immune system, strong bones, teeth and nails, eyesight, fuelling rapid foetal growth, muscle contractions, including heartbeat*

Roasted Lamb with spinach, Almonds and Prunes

This meal is so easy to make and the stuffing adds a wonderful flavour to the lamb. Iron, calcium and essential fatty acids are vital nutrients for pregnancy. They are especially important during the second trimester as your blood volume increases, baby's bones begin to harden and everything else is growing rapidly. Our spinach, almond and prune stuffing provides all of these nutrients and many more. Many women find the need for a little extra fibre during the second trimester and this recipe should help you on your way. Serve with steamed greens and roast vegetables of your choice.

2 x 150 g (5 oz) boneless lamb roast rounds

½ cup pitted prunes, roughly chopped

1 cup baby spinach leaves, roughly chopped

⅓ cup almonds, roughly chopped

1 clove garlic, finely chopped

1 tbs fresh mint leaves

1 tbs lemon juice

Preheat oven to 200°C/400°F. Line a baking tray with baking paper.

Sit the lamb on its flattest edge and make this its base. We now need to create a pocket to hold our stuffing securely within the lamb during cooking. Slice across the longest length of the fillet, leaving 2-cm (¾-inch) at both ends uncut. Now give the pocket some depth and cut about halfway down into the fillet, being careful not to cut through to the base. Repeat procedure on the remaining roast fillet.

Mix the prunes, spinach, almonds, garlic, mint and lemon juice in a bowl. Divide mixture in half and, using clean hands, firmly push the stuffing into the lamb pockets. The ingredients will reduce in volume during cooking so pack as much in as you can. Close and secure the lamb with some cooking string to prevent the stuffing from spilling out in the oven. The meat will also shrink during cooking, with a natural tendency to push the stuffing out, so make sure the pockets are firmly closed. Use four lengths of string and tightly tie around the length and width of the roast.

Transfer lamb to prepared baking tray. Lightly baste with olive oil and season with black pepper. Bake for 20–25 minutes. Remove from the oven, loosely cover with foil and rest the meat in a warm place for 5 minutes. Remove cooking string and slice each roast.

 You should always rest your meat after cooking. This allows the cooking juices to settle and tenderise the meat.

GOOD SOURCE OF: *protein, iron, vitamins B12, B6, C, E and K, calcium, omega 3, folate, potassium, magnesium, phosphorus, selenium, antioxidants*

GOOD FOR MOTHER: *constipation, anaemia, maintaining blood sugar levels, leg cramps, skin elasticity, healthy blood supply, dental problems, calcium function*

GOOD FOR BABY: *manufacture of genetic material and red blood cells, development of strong bone and cell structure, formation of major organs*

Mediterranean Steak with Crunchy Potatoes

Rosemary takes a leading role in both the marinade and potatoes in this meal. This aromatic herb has many health benefits that are useful during pregnancy. It is also said to counteract any harmful substances that may be produced when chargrilling meats. This marinade can be used for steaks generally. For maximum nutritional absorption, serve this meal with a tomato salad (see recipe) or lightly steam broccoli.

2 x 100 g (3½ oz) pieces of lean steak

(fillet, point end rump, New York cuts)

marinade:

3 tbs olive oil

2 tbs balsamic vinegar

1 bay leaf

2 garlic cloves, crushed

½ tsp dried thyme

1 tbs fresh rosemary, chopped

crunchy potatoes:

6–8 small new potatoes

1 tbs olive oil

1 small garlic clove, crushed

1 tsp lemon zest

1 tbs fresh rosemary leaves,

finely chopped

cracked black pepper

143

Whisk all marinade ingredients together in a large bowl. Trim steaks of visible fat and add to the marinade. Rub marinade into steaks. Cover and refrigerate for at least one hour.

Preheat oven to 200°C/400°F to cook the potatoes. Line a baking tray with baking paper.

Cook whole potatoes in a saucepan of boiling water for 8–10 minutes, or until just tender.

Drain and turn out on to a chopping board. Gently crush the potatoes with the back of a spoon or fork. The idea here is to slightly split the potato skin and break up the starch content. When the potatoes are baked, the skins will turn golden crunchy and the insides will be light and fluffy.

Use the warm saucepan you cooked the potatoes in and combine olive oil, garlic, lemon zest and rosemary leaves and season with lots of cracked black pepper. Whisk together and then add potatoes. Gently shake the saucepan and coat the potatoes.

Pour out on to a roasting pan and bake for 25 minutes, or until golden brown. Turn potatoes occasionally to brown evenly and shake the pan to prevent sticking.

Cook steaks to your liking on a preheated barbeque grill. Serve with crunchy potatoes, a tomato salad or steamed broccoli for a complete and balanced meal.

tip *If you don't have time to marinate the steaks, try this quick dry rub marinade. Combine 1 tbs fresh rosemary, 1 tsp dried thyme leaves (or 2 tsp fresh if you have them), 1 clove garlic, 1 tsp lemon rind, cracked black pepper. Rub into lightly oiled steaks.*

GOOD SOURCE OF: *iron, protein, carbohydrates, vitamins B2, B3, B12 and C, calcium, fibre*

GOOD FOR MOTHER: *fatigue, red blood cell production/anaemia, digestion, healthy heart, circulation, increasing blood supply*

GOOD FOR BABY: *manufacture of genetic material and cells, fuelling foetal growth*

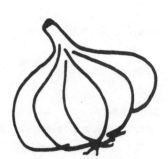

Pork with Mango Salsa

As mentioned before, a colourful dish means lots of different nutrients are being consumed. The vitamin C-rich mango salsa aids the absorption of iron in the pork and promotes soft, supple skin that will stretch without tearing as your belly grows. Despite its name, it is the tearing not the stretching that causes stretch marks.

4 medium butterfly pork steaks

1 large sweet potato, roughly chopped into small cubes

⅓ cup (80 ml/2¾ fl oz) low-fat milk

cracked black pepper

200 g (7 oz) green beans

mango salsa (see recipe page 227)

Trim pork of any white visible fat. Heat barbeque or grill.

Boil sweet potato for 10 minutes, or until tender. Strain and mash with the milk and black pepper. Set aside and keep warm while you lightly steam the beans.

Arrange sweet potato mash in the middle of the serving plates, top with pork fillet, followed by the mango salsa.

Serve the pork and salsa with sweet potato mash and green beans for a nutritionally balanced meal.

145

GOOD SOURCE OF: *rotein, iron, vitamins A, C, E, B1 and B2, folate, fibre*

GOOD FOR MOTHER: *fatigue, digestion, constipation, skin elasticity, converting food to fuel, diabetes, strengthening immune system and blood vessels, dental problems, healthy blood*

GOOD FOR BABY: *eyesight, hardening of bones, formation of muscles, skin and body fat*

Pork Medallions with Nashi Pear, Parmesan and Rocket Salad

This recipe is recommended for those experiencing reflux or heartburn. Rocket is excellent for digestion, as is the nashi pear. Nashi pears are quite neutral in flavour but are incredibly juicy and cleansing to the palate. They can be substituted for regular pears if desired.

1 x 400 g (14 oz) pork fillet

1 tsp olive oil

½ tsp whole fennel seeds

½ tsp ground ginger

1 nashi pear

½ cup shaved parmesan

large handful baby rocket leaves

½ cup walnuts

dressing:

2 tbs extra virgin olive oil or grape seed oil

1 tbs cider vinegar

cracked black pepper

Preheat grill or barbeque. Combine all dressing ingredients and shake or whisk.

Remove any visible fat from the pork and baste with the olive oil.

Slightly grind the fennels seeds to release flavour. Combine with the ginger and rub into the pork.

Place all salad ingredients in a large salad bowl and toss together.

Grill or barbeque the pork for approximately 5 minutes on each side, or until cooked through, turning the fillet only once. Dress the salad and serve with the pork.

tip *The fennel and rocket salad is another perfect accompaniment to barbeque pork.*

GOOD SOURCE OF: *protein, thiamine, folate, vitamins A, D, C and B12, calcium, magnesium, beta-carotene, fibre, essential fatty acids*

GOOD FOR MOTHER: *digestive problems, fatigue, anaemia, healthy blood and haemoglobin production*

GOOD FOR BABY: *providing building blocks and fuel for proper foetal growth, strong bones, teeth and nails*

Tofu and vegetable stir-fry

Iron and protein intake is an important factor in the vegetarian diet during pregnancy. This dish combines the complete protein source, tofu, with vitamin C-rich vegetables to maximise the absorption. This is an easy and delicious dish with loads of vegies, therapeutic spices and sesame seeds for added calcium.

200 g (7 oz) firm tofu

⅓ cup (80 ml/2¾ fl oz) water or vegetable stock

1 tbs tamari (wheat-free soy sauce)

1 tbs oyster sauce

2 tsp sesame seeds

2 tbs canola oil

2 shallots, chopped

2 garlic cloves, finely chopped

2 tsp ginger, finely chopped

1 tsp red chilli, finely chopped

½ red capsicum, sliced in thin strips

1 cup broccoli, cut into small florets

1 cup cauliflower, cut into small florets

½ bunch garlic chives, cut into 3 cm lengths

1 cup snow peas, sugar snap peas or green beans, cut into 3 cm lengths

½ bunch fresh coriander

Cut the tofu into bite-sized cubes and stand on a paper towel to remove excess moisture. Combine water, soy and oyster sauces.

Heat the wok and dry-toast the sesame seeds for 30–60 seconds, or until just golden. The seeds will continue cooking when removed from the heat so be careful not to over-brown. Pour into a small dish and set aside.

147

Heat 1 tsp oil in a hot wok. Add tofu and brown all sides. Be aware that the tofu will splatter a little on contact with the oil due to its high water content. Remove tofu from the wok and drain on paper towel.

Heat 1 tsp remaining oil, this time over a medium-high heat. Add shallots, garlic, ginger and chilli. Stir-fry for 1–2 minutes. Add water and sauces and cook for another 30 seconds before adding all vegetables with the exception of the snow or sugar snap peas. Coat vegetables with the sauces and then return the tofu to the pan. Place a lid on the wok and allow the ingredients to steam for 1–2 minutes.

Remove the lid, add snow peas and stir-fry for one final minute. Stir through coriander and remove wok from heat. Divide into serving bowls, sprinkle with toasted sesame seeds and serve with steamed rice.

GOOD SOURCE OF: *iron, protein, calcium, magnesium, potassium, phosphorus, vitamins A, C, E and B-group including folate, fibre*

GOOD FOR MOTHER: *vegetarians, healthy blood, anaemia, fatigue, skin elasticity, constipation, circulation, hypertension, healthy uterus and placenta, immunity*

GOOD FOR BABY: *functioning of all organs, healthy cell growth, development of eyes, skin and nervous system, strong bones and teeth*

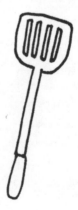

Banana Baby Cheesecakes

A delicious low-fat treat. Ricotta cheese is safe to eat when cooked, although it is advised to use the packaged ricotta rather than the fresh variety sold in delis as there is much less chance of contamination. But can I say, you must try this recipe with fresh ricotta when not pregnant as it is simply heaven!

2 eggs

500 g (1 lb) low-fat ricotta

⅓ cup skim milk powder

2 tbs self-raising flour

1 tsp vanilla extract, or seeds of 1 vanilla bean

1 tbs honey

3 bananas

Preheat oven to 160°C/325°F. Use a 6 x deep-case muffin tin and line each case with baking paper.

Beat eggs until light and fluffy. Add the ricotta, skim milk powder, flour, vanilla and honey and blend to form a smooth paste.

In a large mixing bowl, mash bananas to a smooth consistency. Add the ricotta mixture and use a large metal spoon to gently fold ingredients together. Spoon the mixture evenly into the muffin cases, filling no more than ¾ of the case.

Bake for 25–30 minutes, or until cheesecakes have set. To test, gently tap the centre of the cheesecakes for firmness. Remove from oven and cool the cheesecakes in the tray. Chill for one hour prior to serving. Makes 6.

tip *Store cheesecakes in the fridge in an airtight container lined with a paper towel for up to 2–3 days. Also suitable for freezing. Purchase vanilla extract rather than essence—there is a big difference. Essence contains chemicals that are not desired in any diet.*

GOOD SOURCE OF: *potassium, magnesium, vitamin B, calcium, protein*

GOOD FOR MOTHER: *healthy skin, blood pressure, leg cramps*

GOOD FOR BABY: *brain and spinal development, steady heartbeat, healthy teeth, muscle contractions and nerve function and their coordination, strong bones*

Mango with Passionfruit and Yoghurt

This recipe is super rich in vitamin C, which is fabulous for toning and maintaining a healthy uterus in preparation for childbirth. This nutrient also promotes the production of collagen to make skin more elastic and less inclined to tear and produce stretch marks as your body grows. Meanwhile, your baby is growing its own healthy skin, hair, bones, nails, teeth and gums and is developing great eyesight.

All this from one yummy dessert!

2 mangoes

2 passionfruit

1 cup low-fat yoghurt

Cross-hatch the flesh of the mangoes and scoop out into serving bowls.

Scoop the seeds of the passionfruit over the mangos and top with your favourite low-fat yoghurt. Plain or vanilla go well with this recipe.

GOOD SOURCE OF: *vitamins A, C and E, calcium, protein, iron, potassium, fibre*

GOOD FOR MOTHER: *immune system, healthy skin, teeth and bones, skin elasticity, toning and preparing uterus for birth, constipation, hypertension, bleeding gums and dental problems*

GOOD FOR BABY: *promoting cell growth, eyesight, muscle/nerve impulses including heartbeat*

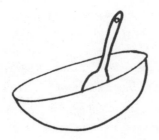

white Peach and Raspberry Trifle

This is a modern, low-fat take on the traditional trifle dessert. The light, fresh flavours make this a fabulous finale to any summer barbeque or dinner party. Seasonal sweet white peaches teamed with antioxidant-rich raspberries and the goodness of yoghurt dish up a dessert that is deliciously good for you. White nectarines or mixed berries can be used as substitutes.

1 cup (250 ml/8 fl oz) low-fat plain or vanilla yoghurt

½ cup (125 ml/4 fl oz) freshly squeezed orange juice

2 tbs honey

4 ripe white peaches

1 packet Italian sponge fingers

2 cups raspberries, fresh or defrosted

½ cup slivered almonds, lightly toasted

151

Combine yoghurt, orange juice and honey and mix until honey has dissolved. Wash peaches thoroughly. De-seed and slice the peaches, leaving the skin on.

Use a medium serving bowl and cover the base with a single layer of sponge fingers. You may need to break the sponge fingers to fit the shape of the bowl. Cover the sponge fingers with one third of the yoghurt mixture. Layer with half of the raspberries and half of the sliced peaches.

Repeat layering sequence with biscuits, yoghurt, remaining raspberries and peaches. Finally, top with remaining yoghurt and half of the slivered almonds.

Cover the trifle with a piece of greaseproof or baking paper and lightly press down with your hands to compact the trifle. Press the baking paper against the inside edges of the bowl to seal and cover with aluminium foil. Once again, press down lightly to compact the trifle layers.

Refrigerate for 3 hours or overnight. Sprinkle with remaining slivered almonds to serve.

tip *Individual trifles can be made for an impressive dinner party dessert. Break the sponge fingers to fit the base of the serving dishes or glasses and layer trifle ingredients as in the recipe above.*

GOOD SOURCE OF: *calcium, protein, vitamins B12, C and D, magnesium, phosphorus, potassium*

GOOD FOR MOTHER: *digestion, fatigue, immunity, healthy skin and hair, nourishing the uterus, lactation*

GOOD FOR BABY: *providing building blocks for baby's bones, teeth and nails, eyesight, development of nervous system, regulating heartbeat*

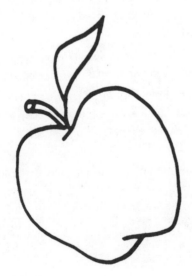

Guilt-free Plum Pastries

This dessert won't send blood sugar levels soaring. Plums are low GI and contain powerful antioxidants to keep you strong and healthy. They are also excellent for healthy liver function. The liver works very hard during the second and third trimesters to support, cleanse and filter the increased blood supply necessary to maintain the pregnancy. It is also thought that cinnamon helps to regulate normal blood sugar levels.

> ½ cup (125 ml/4 fl oz) orange juice
>
> ½ tsp ground cinnamon
>
> 3–4 plums
>
> 1 sheet of fat-reduced puff pastry

Preheat the oven to 180°C/350°F.

Place the orange juice and cinnamon in a shallow bowl and whisk to combine. Thinly slice the plums and place in the orange juice. Toss to coat the plums and marinate for 5 minutes or so.

Line a baking tray with a sheet of baking paper, slightly larger than your puff pastry. Place the pastry sheet on the baking paper and defrost. Cut the pastry sheet into quarters for four even squares. Separate the pastry squares slightly. Arrange the plums evenly on top of the pastry, leaving a 2 cm border edge free of fruit. Baste the edges with the remaining orange juice and drizzle any excess over the plums. Bake for 20 minutes, or until pastry edges puff up and turn golden brown.

Serve warm with a generous dollop of your favourite yoghurt. Makes 4.

 tip *Plums can be substituted for other stone fruit varieties such as apricots, peaches or nectarines. Thinly sliced apples, pears or mixed berries are also delicious.*

GOOD SOURCE OF: *fibre, potassium, antioxidants*

GOOD FOR MOTHER: *aiding liver function, constipation, digestion, hypertension, lowering cholesterol, diabetes*

GOOD FOR BABY: *normal development of the central nervous system, protecting body tissue and cells*

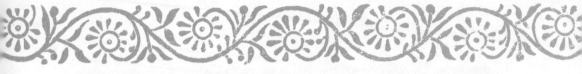

Third Trimester weeks 29 to Birth

This is the trimester where you should gain the most weight. Your body is preparing for childbirth and your baby is growing rapidly. Now is the time to slightly increase the kilojoules with smart choices of high-fibre complex carbohydrates, protein and lots of fresh vegetables.

Good nutrition is important throughout pregnancy, but it is vital to continue the good work in the final phase. This is when the more serious complications can arise, but most can be completely avoided by eating a wholesome diet. Remember, a healthy pregnancy diet aids postnatal recovery.

Calcium intake continues to be important. The baby accumulates the majority of its calcium for strong teeth and bones in the third trimester. Omega 3 and iodine are essential for the rapid brain development of the foetus.

Tiredness and fatigue may return due to difficulties in sleeping and the sheer burden of carrying your fully-grown baby. Digestive problems are also a main complaint. This is due to the expanding uterus which squishes your stomach to a much smaller capacity. Snacks and smaller meals five to six times a day are the key to a more comfortable final trimester.

As your pregnancy comes to an end, you may find you have more time on your hands. Those who work may have commenced maternity leave; others will be winding down. This is a great opportunity to prepare for those first few days, weeks and even months, of motherhood by cooking and freezing meals in advance.

The essential nutrients needed at this time are: calcium, magnesium, omega 3, iodine, iron, B-group vitamins (folate and B12), zinc.

Progression of Baby

WHAT'S HAPPENING	WHAT'S NEEDED
Baby gains most weight and moves about more frequently	complex carbohydrates, protein, folate
Most rapid brain development (under-nourishment can prevent optimal brain development)	omega 3, zinc, iodine, complex carbohydrates
Lungs develop and mature	calcium

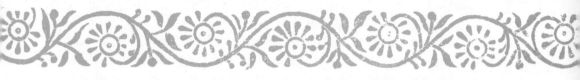

Nervous and immune systems begin functioning	zinc, omega 3, folate, protein, vitamins B6 and C
Begins to manufacture own red blood cells, produce own blood supply and lay down iron stores	iron, folate, vitamins B12 and B5
Hair, skin and fat covers body	zinc, selenium, B-group vitamins
Teeth and nails develop	calcium, magnesium

Progression of mother

WHAT'S HAPPENING	WHAT'S NEEDED
Most weight gained and kilojoules needed	
Body prepares for birth	vitamin C, zinc to tone the uterus
Colostrum is produced for breastfeeding	calcium, vitamin C, essential fatty acids
Blood volume peaks between weeks 28–30	iron, folate, vitamins B12 and B5

Common complaints of the third trimester

- Tiredness/fatigue (see page 46)
- Dental problems (see page 50)
- Anaemia (see page 97)
- Digestive problems (see page 98)
- Fluid retention (see page 101)
- Leg cramps (see page 101)
- Stretch marks (see page 102)

Gestational Diabetes

Gestational diabetes is a form of diabetes, or high blood glucose levels, that develops during pregnancy. It is usually a temporary condition, with most cases detected around weeks 28 to 30. All expectant mothers should be tested for it around this time.

Diabetes generally is on the increase in today's society. Gestational diabetes is also a growing concern, with the condition being diagnosed in up to 9 per cent of pregnancies and rising. The good news is that it can be completely avoided and managed by a balanced diet and regular exercise.

Gestational diabetes occurs because glucose tolerance decreases as pregnancy progresses. Hormones produced by the placenta prevent insulin acting efficiently, so the body needs to produce more insulin than usual. Insulin removes glucose from the bloodstream. If inefficient, glucose will remain in the blood for longer, causing blood sugar levels to rise. This can cause complications for both mother and baby.

The condition does usually subside after delivery, but it can increase the mother's risk of developing diabetes later in life by up to 50 per cent.

There are also implications to the baby. High glucose levels are passed directly from the mother's bloodstream to the baby, who will produce (and be born with) extra insulin to cope with the excess glucose. Insulin is the most potent growth hormone known to man. The baby will grow *very* fast and *very* big. Larger babies are generally harder to deliver. The baby may also be born with a low blood glucose condition known as hypoglycemia, which can continue throughout its life.

In more serious cases, diabetes can damage the placenta, result in kidney failure and premature or stillborn births. Symptoms include excessive thirst, fatigue and passing large amounts of urine.

Diet and regular exercise can prevent gestational diabetes and are effective treatments if the condition does develop. The main objective is to keep blood glucose levels in a healthy range.

Tips to avoid gestational diabetes from the very beginning of your pregnancy:

- limit your sugar intake to a minimum
- avoid processed foods
- control salt intake and do not add salt to foods
- eat no more than 3 to 4 servings of fruit per day
- eat more whole plant foods and wholegrain foods
- stick to low GI choices when selecting complex carbohydrates
- eat low-fat dairy products.

A diet high in carbohydrates can cause an increase in glucose levels. If you are considered to be at a high risk for developing gestational diabetes you will need to monitor your carbohydrate intake. Seek advice from your health practitioner if unsure.

High risk factors include:

- having a family history of diabetes

- being overweight

- being over 30 years old

- having had gestational diabetes in a previous pregnancy or being of Aboriginal, Asian, Pacific Islander or Indian descent.

Recent studies have shown that half a teaspoon of cinnamon daily for 40 days significantly lowered and maintained blood sugar levels in a group of Type 2 diabetic volunteers.

HyPeRtension anD PRe-ecLamPsia

Hypertension (or high blood pressure) can interfere with foetal growth and the proper functioning of the placenta, which supplies blood and oxygen to your baby. Hypertension can also contribute to fluid retention, cause kidney failure and make the liver and heart work harder. Serious cases of high blood pressure can lead to pre-eclampsia, a poisoning of the blood and a high risk factor for placental abruption, premature birth or forced pre-term delivery.

Pre-eclampsia is a very dangerous condition. It is rarely diagnosed prior to week 20, but regular blood pressure check-ups are advisable. If a condition does develop, the mother is admitted to hospital for observation. If untreated, it can progress to eclampsia, when often the only real cure is pre-term delivery or termination of the pregnancy.

Symptoms of pre-eclampsia include:

- sudden weight gain

- swollen ankles

- protein in urine

- obesity

- diabetes

- headaches/dizziness.

Thankfully, diet is the most effective way of controlling hypertension. Dairy products and fresh fruit and vegetables can help to lower blood pressure. Lack of protein, zinc, vitamin C and E deficiencies and general poor nutrition have been linked to high blood pressure. Too much salt in the diet can also be a contributing factor.

Obesity and diabetes are high risk factors of hypertension, so exercise and steady weight gain are important factors in controlling blood pressure. Food aids for high blood pressure:

- apple, watermelon, mango, orange
- carrot, celery, beetroot, spinach, parsley, cucumber
- onions, garlic.

To avoid hypertension, make sure your diet includes the following:

- loads of fresh fruit and vegetables (8 to 10 servings per day, with no more than 4 servings of fruit)
- vitamin C
- vitamin E—vegetable oils, nuts and seeds, wheat, avocado
- omega 3—fish
- first class protein foods—lean meat
- foods rich in calcium—low-fat dairy products
- magnesium—wheatgerm, brazil nuts, almonds, pumpkin and sesame seeds
- potassium—low-fat dairy, fresh fruit and vegetables, chickpeas and lentils.

Varicose veins

Varicose veins can be hereditary but can also be triggered by excess weight and pressure on the legs. To reduce your risk, exercise regularly to encourage good blood circulation and take some pressure off by raising your legs when sitting. Follow a high-fibre diet as constipation and forced bowel movements puts added pressure on the veins.

Food aids for varicose veins:

- high-fibre diet
- vitamin C—believed to keep veins healthy and elastic
- buckwheat and its products, such as bread, flour and soba noodles.

Sleeplessness

Sleeplessness is likely to be experienced towards the end of pregnancy simply because the sheer size of your belly makes it hard to get comfortable and sleep at night. Calcium and magnesium are natural sedatives, so eating rich food sources at night may assist. A banana smoothie is a perfect example (see *Calcium* and *Magnesium*). Complex carbohydrates also tend to bring on drowsiness, as can a glass of milk or chamomile tea. Try one of my healthy muffins and a warm milk or cup of herbal tea before bedtime.

✿ recipes for third trimester
weeks 29 to Birth

Scrambled Eggs with Mushroom and Asparagus Parcels

Scrambled eggs must be the quickest way to prepare eggs. They take less time to cook than a boiled egg and less preparation than a poached one. I have used cottage cheese as a healthy alternative to cream to create a creamy consistency. The cottage cheese melts during cooking to achieve a similar result. The health benefits of this dish are incredible, especially when teamed up with the mushrooms and asparagus. Enjoy for general good health.

3 tsp balsamic vinegar

2 tsp extra virgin olive oil

¼ tsp dried thyme

1 tbs fresh parsley, chopped

cracked black pepper

½ clove garlic (optional)

6–8 mushrooms

4 asparagus spears

2 eggs, preferably biodynamic

½ cup low-fat cottage cheese

2 slices wholegrain toast

160

Combine the vinegar, one teaspoon of the oil, thyme, parsley, pepper and garlic in a bowl. Add the mushrooms and asparagus and coat with the marinade. Pour the mixture on to a sheet of aluminium foil, large enough to securely parcel the mushrooms and asparagus. Fold the sides together to make a parcel and firmly secure the joins to ensure the marinade does not seep out during cooking.

Heat a non-stick frying pan over a medium heat and place the mushroom parcel into the dry pan. The heat from the pan will steam the vegetables. Cook for 3 minutes. Use a pair of tongs to move and gently shake the parcels occasionally to prevent the mixture from sticking to the foil. Remove the parcel from the pan and keep sealed until ready to serve.

Break the eggs into a bowl and lightly whisk. Add the cottage cheese and black pepper and whisk until combined and a smooth consistency.

Ensure the pan is of only a medium heat. It is important to not brown the eggs if we are to achieve a creamy consistency. Add the remaining teaspoon of oil and swirl around to coat the pan. The eggs will only take a minute or so to cook, so work quickly. Use a non-metal spatula or wooden spoon and push and fold eggs toward the centre of the pan, scooping the cooked eggs on top of each other. Turn the heat off as soon as the eggs are JUST cooked and keep scrambling for another 15–20 seconds. The eggs will continue to cook with the heat of the pan, so be sure to serve almost immediately to avoid over-cooked eggs.

Pile scrambled eggs on top of the toast and open the mushroom parcel, tipping the vegetables on to the plate along with the cooking juices. Sprinkle the eggs with some fresh chives, thyme leaves or parsley. Serves 1.

tip *For successful scrambled eggs, always use fresh eggs and a good quality non-stick frying pan. Eggs take just minutes to scramble, so have all other ingredients prepared before you start cooking. For an even quicker version, sprinkle scrambled eggs with a little paprika and serve with a handful of baby rocket leaves instead of the mushrooms. Ready in 5 minutes. The mushroom and asparagus parcels are great with cottage cheese on wholegrain toast.*

GOOD SOURCE OF: *protein, iron, iodine, omega 3, vitamins A, C, D and B-group including folate and B12, calcium, selenium, fibre, phosphorus, potassium*

GOOD FOR MOTHER: *anaemia, fatigue, skin elasticity, strengthening blood vessels, boosting immune system, protecting against cell damage, increased nutritional absorption, production of red blood cells, body cells and genetic material*

GOOD FOR BABY: *development of all major organs, brain and central nervous system, healthy skin and eyes, strong bones, fuelling foetal growth*

Berry Compote

This is a healthy version of jam on toast, with no added sugar or preservatives—just the amazing natural goodness and sweetness of berries. It can be served warm or cold and is delicious with yoghurt or porridge as other breakfast alternatives. It also doubles as a very impressive dessert over, dare I suggest, ice-cream!

1½ cups frozen mixed berries

1 tsp balsamic vinegar

2 slices light rye sourdough

low-fat cottage cheese or cream cheese to serve

Defrost the berries and place in a small saucepan with the balsamic vinegar.

Gently simmer over a medium heat for 2–3 minutes, continually stirring as the berries soften to form a gorgeous thick sauce. Remove from heat and cool slightly in the saucepan.

162

Lightly toast sourdough. Spread with cottage or cream cheese and then spoon the berries and sauce on top. Simply divine. Serves 1.

GOOD SOURCE OF: *antioxidants, vitamins A, C, E and B-group, fibre, calcium*

GOOD FOR MOTHER: *maintaining health of all major organs especially the heart and kidneys, hypertension, fatigue, circulation, varicose veins, repairing tissues and wounds, nourishing placenta and uterus, lactation, immunity*

GOOD FOR BABY: *eyesight, healthy cells, skin, bones, teeth and gums*

Mixed Grain Porridge

Wholegrains are one of the best sources of the B-group vitamins and are a complex carbohydrate. These nutrients are vital during the third trimester to fuel your baby's rapid growth and energy needs. By mixing the three grains in this porridge, a wider range of nutrients is consumed. Barley, for instance, is rich in calcium and potassium. This is a warming and comforting breakfast during the winter months. If you have been enjoying the mixed grain natural muesli, this is a great winter alternative.

⅓ cup each of rolled barley and rolled oats

½ cup rolled rye (for gluten-free version use rolled barley and rice flakes)

1 cup (250 ml/8 fl oz) water

½ cup (125 ml/4 fl oz) low-fat milk/soy milk

4 pitted prunes, chopped

1 tbs LSA

1 banana

milk to serve

163

Place grains, water, milk and prunes in a small saucepan. Bring porridge to the boil, stirring constantly to prevent the grains sticking to the pan. Reduce to medium heat and continue stirring until almost all the liquid has been absorbed and you have a creamy consistency.

Remove from heat and spoon porridge into a serving bowl. Sprinkle with LSA and sliced banana and serve with additional warm milk if desired. Serves 1.

GOOD SOURCE OF: *calcium, magnesium, protein, B-group vitamins, fibre, essential fatty acids*

GOOD FOR MOTHER: *constipation, excellent energy source, gestational diabetes, heartburn and reflux, dental problems, leg cramps, kidney function, hypertension*

GOOD FOR BABY: *strong bone structure, fuelling foetal growth, development of brain, lungs and central nervous system, growth of skin, hair, teeth and body fat, muscle contractions*

Salmon, Leek and Thyme Omelette

This recipe combines the unbeatable goodness of both eggs and salmon. These two foods provide nutrients that are absolutely fantastic for foetal brain development, toning and nourishing the uterus and reducing the risk of pre-term birth. Enjoy this meal for breakfast, lunch or dinner, knowing you are doing the absolute best for your baby and yourself.

1 tbs olive oil

½ cup leeks, white parts only, finely sliced

1 x 110 g (4 oz) can red salmon

2 shallots, finely chopped

1 tsp dried thyme or 1 tbs fresh thyme leaves

cracked black pepper

2 eggs

2 tbs water

½ cup grated cheese, tasty or parmesan

Heat olive oil over medium heat in a non-stick frying pan. Add leeks and cook gently for 5 minutes or until soft. Transfer to a mixing bowl and combine with salmon, shallots and thyme. Season to taste with black pepper.

Break eggs into a separate bowl, add 2 tablespoons of water and whisk until combined.

Wipe the pan clean with some paper towel and if your pan needs oil to prevent sticking, heat a little extra olive oil. Add eggs, swirling pan to evenly cover the base and allowing the uncooked eggs to flow out to the sides. Cook for 1 minute, then add leek and salmon mixture in the centre of the omelette and top with cheese, leaving a 2 cm edge on the omelette with no filling.

Cook until egg mixture just sets. Fold omelette in half and gently slide out of the pan on to a serving plate. Serve immediately on top of wholegrain toast.

tip *Try these alternative fillings: canned tuna, red capsicum, red onion and fresh parsley; or Baby spinach leaves, sliced mushrooms and tasty cheese.*

GOOD SOURCE OF: *essential fatty acids, zinc, protein, iodine, vitamins D and B-group, folate, calcium*

GOOD FOR MOTHER: *reducing risk of pre-term labour and osteoporosis, preparation of uterus for birth, fatigue, anaemia, fluid retention, skin elasticity, healthy blood, leg cramps, production of colostrum and reproductive hormones, lactation*

GOOD FOR BABY: *rapid brain development, maturation of lungs, hardening of teeth and bones, eyesight, functioning of nervous and immune systems, manufacture of baby's own red blood cells and blood supply, final development stages of hair, skin, teeth, nails and fat*

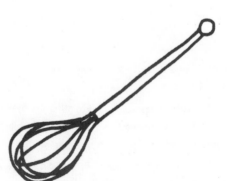

Salmon and Egg Salad

This is the perfect lunch to take and make at work. Pack a can of salmon, an unpeeled boiled egg, a whole lemon and some uncut veges in a lunch box and refrigerate until meal time. It takes just 5 minutes to throw together.

½ avocado, sliced

125 g (4½ oz) can salmon slices in olive oil

½ punnet grape tomatoes, halved

2 shallots, finely sliced

small handful of sugar snap peas, stalks and string removed

a handful of watercress or baby spinach leaves, roughly chopped

1 boiled egg, peeled and cut into quarters

fresh mint leaves, shredded

juice of 1 lemon

Place all ingredients, with the exception of the lemon, in a medium-sized serving bowl. Gently toss to combine ingredients. Season with black pepper and a good squeeze of fresh lemon juice. Serves 1.

tip *A sprinkle of sesame seeds is a nice addition. This salad also makes a yummy filling for a bread roll, wrap or even rice paper rolls. For a gourmet twist, flake hot smoked ocean trout or chargrilled salmon fillet through this salad instead of canned salmon. Sprinkle with sesame seeds and drizzle with lemon soy dressing. Perfect for Sunday lunch with friends.*

GOOD SOURCE OF: *omega 3, protein, calcium, iron, zinc, iodine, potassium, folate, vitamins A, C, D and B12*

GOOD FOR MOTHER: *fatigue, dental and digestive problems, gestational diabetes, healthy heart and blood, nourishing uterus and placenta, regulating body temperature, skin elasticity, production of colostrum, lactation, hypertension*

GOOD FOR BABY: *development of brain, lungs and nervous system, eyesight, strong bones, teeth and nails, growth of hair, skin and body fat, baby's blood supply and iron stores*

Sesame Salmon with Crisp Asian Salad

You should enjoy a comfortable pregnancy with this recipe. It is nutritionally rich, with ingredients combined to bring out the best in each other. It also provides everything needed to support the rapid foetal growth and brain development of the third trimester. The benefits of salmon are well-known, with sesame seeds providing an extra boost of calcium. This is a light, cleansing dish that will satisfy without causing digestive discomforts. It can be served for lunch or dinner, with a small bowl of steamed rice if desired.

½ lebanese cucumber or 1 stick celery

2 asparagus spears

½ red capsicum

½ green capsicum

2 shallots

½ cup fresh coriander, roughly chopped

2 x 100 g (3½ oz) salmon fillets

1–2 tbs sesame seeds

dressing:

3 tbs lime juice

2 tbs fish sauce

1 tbs honey

167

Preheat the grill to a medium heat.

First, make your salad. Note that all vegetables are served raw. Thinly slice vegetables into approximately 3–4 cm lengths to resemble long matchsticks. It seems to complement the crunchy texture that we are after and they look fabulous all cut the same length. Place in a medium-size bowl with the coriander. Toss ingredients together to mix well.

Make the dressing by combining the lime juice, fish sauce and honey in a small bowl. Whisk until the honey has dissolved. Do not dress the salad yet.

Lightly brush the skinless side of the salmon fillets with a little olive oil. Pour the sesame seeds out on to a plate or chopping board and press the skinless side of the salmon into the seeds to form a nice crust, using as many seeds as you need.

Place the salmon on a grill tray and grill for 8–10 minutes, depending on the thickness of the fillet. The sesame seeds will be slightly toasted. Remove the fillets as soon as they are just cooked and place on to serving plates. Remember, fish continues to cook for a few minutes after it has been removed from the heat source. Drizzle a little of the dressing over each fillet, probably 1 teaspoon for each fillet. Pour the remaining dressing over the salad.

Divide the Asian salad evenly between the two plates to accompany the salmon.

tip *For a complete change of cuisine, serve the sesame salmon fillet with a simple salad of baby rocket leaves, shallots and fresh tomato. Drizzle the salad and salmon with a dash of balsamic vinegar.*

GOOD SOURCE OF: *protein, iron, omega 3, vitamins A, B12, C, K and E, zinc, iodine, calcium, folate*

GOOD FOR MOTHER: *anaemia, healthy blood, skin, liver, kidneys and heart, hypertension, dental problems, constipation, fluid retention, leg cramps, nourishing uterus, lactation*

GOOD FOR BABY: *development of brain, lungs, hair, skin and body fat, promoting and protecting healthy body cells, strong bones, teeth and nails, functioning of nervous and immune systems, eyesight, building baby's iron stores*

168

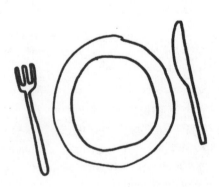

Bara-Burger with Babaganoush

If you are not mad on either eating or cooking fish, this might be the recipe for you. I suggest using baby barramundi as the smaller fillets are more suitable for a burger and have lower levels of mercury, making it a safe pregnancy choice. Baby barramundi is usually sold as a whole fish, so ask your fishmonger to fillet and remove all scales and skin from the fish for you.

1 zucchini

1 small red capsicum

2 wholegrain bread rolls

babaganoush to serve

1 baby barramundi, filleted

handful of baby rocket or spinach leaves

Preheat oven grill to a medium-high heat. Slice zucchini lengthways in 4 cm length strips. Cut the capsicum in half, remove seeds and pith. Cut the bread rolls in half, leaving one end intact. Place the zucchini and capsicum under a medium-heat grill and cook for 5 minutes, until slightly softened. Slice the capsicum in strips once cooked. Towards the end of cooking, lightly toast the inside of the rolls and then spread both sides generously with babaganoush.

169

Meanwhile, lightly baste fish fillets with olive oil and season with cracked black pepper. Heat a non-stick frying pan and cook fish for 2–3 minutes on one side before turning and cooking for the same time on the other side.

Layer the rocket, zucchini and capsicum on the bread roll spread with babaganoush. Top with the fish fillet and close with the top of the roll.

tip *Herbed yoghurt is also fantastic with fish burgers. Cucumber, tomato and baby spinach leaves are other filling options. Salmon can also be used.*

GOOD SOURCE OF: *omega 3, iodine, zinc, protein, iron, calcium, B-group vitamins including folate and B12, fibre*
GOOD FOR MOTHER: *healthy heart and blood, anaemia, skin elasticity, dental problems, repairing tissues/healing wounds, toning uterus, reducing risk of pre-term birth, red blood cell production of both mother and baby*
GOOD FOR BABY: *aiding brain development and function, growth of hair, skin and body fat, healthy bones, teeth and body cells*

Red Lentil Soup

Lentils are a high quality protein source as they are low in fat, mineral rich and provide sustained energy to fuel foetal growth. They are also a great source of dietary fibre and maintain the general health of the digestive tract. Legumes do have the reputation of causing flatulence or bloating and for this reason are sadly excluded from many diets. This need not be the case. Lentil dishes are usually heavily spiced, which is no coincidence. The spices commonly used, namely cumin, turmeric and coriander, assist digestion and help to minimise and counteract these unpleasant side effects. Another tip to avoid flatulence is to remove the brown foam residue that forms during the cooking process. Scoop this off with a metal spoon throughout the cooking process and you should have minimal after effects.

170

1 carrot, diced

1 stick celery, diced

1 red capsicum, diced

100 g (3½ oz) green beans, diced

1 brown onion, diced

3 cloves garlic, crushed

2 tbs olive oil

1 tsp cumin

2 tsp ground coriander

1 tsp paprika

½ tsp turmeric

4 cups (1 litre/32 fl oz) vegetable stock (salt-reduced if not homemade)

1 cup red lentils, rinsed and drained

½ cup fresh coriander

plain yoghurt as a serving option

Chop and prepare all vegetables. Heat oil over medium heat in a large pot. Add onion and red capsicum and cook for 2–3 minutes. Add garlic and cook for a further minute before adding the spices. Cook for 15 seconds, stirring continuously, and then add one quarter of a cup of the stock to avoid spices sticking to the pan. Stir through lentils, remaining vegetables and stock.

Bring soup to the boil, then cover and reduce heat to simmer for 20–25 minutes, or until lentils are cooked. Stir through fresh coriander and serve with a dollop of plain or herbed yoghurt and a wholegrain roll for a complete protein meal. Serves 4.

tip *This soup will keep in the fridge for 3–4 days, or frozen for 2 months. If you are freezing this soup, do not add coriander until serving.*

GOOD SOURCE OF: *protein, fibre, calcium, iron, magnesium, potassium, phosphorus, vitamins A, B and C, essential fatty acids*

GOOD FOR MOTHER: *vegetarians, diabetes, constipation, digestion, hypertension, healthy blood, anaemia, immunity, iron absorption, nourishing heart, skin elasticity*

GOOD FOR BABY: *strong bones, teeth and nails, healthy skin, development of central nervous system*

171

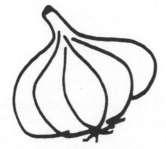

Vegetarian Pita Pizzas

These mini pizzas are the perfect size for a shrinking stomach and provide close to all of the nutrients essential to the third trimester. The hummus is a high-protein calcium source, but if your daily intake has not been met and you are not a vegan, add grated cheese to this recipe. Select from parmesan, cheddar or tasty.

½ punnet cherry tomatoes, halved, or 4 semi-roasted roma tomatoes

4 wholemeal pita bases

hummus, homemade or purchased

1 zucchini, thinly sliced

½ red capsicum, diced

2 marinated artichokes, drained and sliced

½ cup button mushrooms, halved

2 sprigs of fresh rosemary or a handful of parsley

fresh rocket to serve

172

Preheat oven to 170°C/325°F. Grease and line a baking tray.

If slow-roasting tomatoes, cut tomatoes lengthways, drizzle with balsamic vinegar and pepper and place in the oven for 10 minutes, or as long as it takes to prepare pizzas.

Spread pita bases very generously with hummus. This is your protein and calcium source. Arrange zucchini slices, capsicum, artichokes and mushrooms on top of the hummus. Scatter with the tomatoes and fresh herbs.

Bake for 8–10 minutes, or until the zucchini softens. Scatter with fresh rocket leaves to serve. Makes 4.

GOOD SOURCE OF: *protein, calcium, iron, vitamins C and B-group, magnesium, essential fatty acids*

GOOD FOR MOTHER: *vegetarians, fatigue, digestion, circulation, constipation, hypertension, fluid retention, healthy heart and liver*

GOOD FOR BABY: *developing blood supply, nerve and sexual development, growth of organs, hair, skin and body fat*

GRiLLeD SaLmon with GReen Bean and Potato SaLaD

This is a perfectly balanced meal and will help with many of the common complaints of pregnancy as well as facilitate the growth of a very healthy baby. It is especially rich in omega 3, with the dressing adding to the health benefits of our ingredients. You will note the use of grape seed oil rather than olive oil. Grape seed oil is actually the healthier of the two oils. It is also lighter in flavour and will not overpower any of the other ingredients. Garlic is fantastic with seafood as it helps preserve the essential fatty acids found in seafood, and the lemon juice and parsley contains vitamin C to increase iron absorption.

8–10 small chat potatoes

2 x 150g (5 oz) salmon fillets

200 g (7 oz) green beans, halved

½ small red onion, finely diced

½ cup fresh parsley, finely chopped

dressing:

3 tbs grape seed oil

2 tsp lemon juice

1 tsp Dijon mustard

1 tbs parsley or dill

1 small clove garlic, crushed

cracked black pepper

small pinch iodised salt

173

Scrub potato skins clean, pat dry and cut into quarters. Bring a medium saucepan of water to the boil. Add potatoes and cook for 10 minutes, until just tender. Drain.

Prepare dressing by combining all ingredients and vigorously shaking or whisking together.

Preheat oven grill to medium–high heat. Drain potatoes and place under the grill and lightly brown each side—this takes about 15 minutes. The potatoes may seem a little dry at this stage, but they will be moistened with the dressing in the salad.

Place salmon fillets, skin-side down, under the grill with the potatoes. Cook for 7–8 minutes, or until just cooked through.

While salmon and potatoes are cooking, prepare the salad. Wash and trim green beans and cut in half. Steam the beans for 1–2 minutes for a firm/tender crunch. Place into a salad bowl with the onion and parsley. Season with cracked black pepper.

Remove salmon from the grill and place on to serving plates. Add the potatoes to the salad and toss through ½ of the dressing. Drizzle remaining dressing over the salmon fillets and serve with the salad.

GOOD SOURCE OF: *iron, protein, omega 3, zinc, iodine, potassium, calcium, vitamins C and B-group, folate*

GOOD FOR MOTHER: *anaemia, digestion, constipation, hypertension, fatigue, lactation, toning uterus for birth, boosting immune system, production of colostrum, lactation, regulating body temperature, skin elasticity, healthy heart, blood and skin for mother and baby*

GOOD FOR BABY: *development of brain and major organs, functioning of immune and central nervous systems, eyesight, weight gain, manufacture of baby's red blood cells and iron stores*

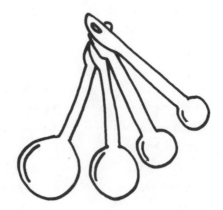

fresh and simple Tuna Pastas

Tuna pasta would have to be one of the most popular and accessible recipes as it suits a busy lifestyle as well as a budget-conscious one. It is also ideal for the pregnancy diet as canned tuna is a fantastic nutritional source and should be a pantry staple. Health authorities have deemed canned tuna safe to eat in regard to its mercury levels; fresh tuna, however, should be avoided. Here are two tuna pasta recipes that I hope will become regulars of your cooking repertoire. Both involve minimal preparation and loads of nutrition and energy.

Tuna Pasta Mediterranean

200 g (7 oz) buckwheat or wholemeal pasta spirals

⅓ cup (80 ml/2¾ fl oz) pasta cooking water

1 tbs olive oil

1 clove garlic, crushed

1 tbs capers, rinsed and drained

¼ cup olives (from a jar rather than a deli counter)

100 g (3½ oz) green beans, cut into 2 cm lengths

1 punnet cherry tomatoes

185 g (6½ oz) can tuna slices in springwater

½ cup fresh parsley or basil, finely chopped

cracked black pepper

175

Cook pasta according to packet directions, until just al dente. The pasta will be cooked again later in the recipe. Drain pasta and reserve ⅓ cup of the cooking water.

Wipe the saucepan with a paper towel to remove all water. This will prevent the oil from spitting when heated. Heat the olive oil over a medium heat. Add garlic and capers and cook for 1–2 minutes, being careful not to burn or brown the garlic as it can turn bitter in taste. Add the olives, beans, tomatoes and pasta water and cook for a further 2 minutes before adding the tuna and pasta. Toss to combine all ingredients and gently warm through for a minute or so.

Stir through herbs just prior to serving and generously season with cracked black pepper.

Tuna Pasta with Rocket and Lemon

150 g (5 oz) wholemeal or buckwheat pasta

1 cup (250 ml/8 fl oz) pasta cooking water

1 clove garlic, crushed

1 tbs capers, rinsed and drained

1 bunch fresh asparagus, trimmed and cut into 3 cm lengths

juice and rind of one lemon

1 x 185 g (6½ oz) can tuna in olive oil, drained

2 large handfuls rocket leaves

parmesan cheese to serve

cracked black pepper

176

Cook pasta according to packet directions until just al dente as the pasta will be cooked for a further few minutes later in the recipe. Drain pasta and reserve 1 cup of the cooking water.

Place ½ cup of the pasta water back into the saucepan. Add garlic, capers and lemon rind and simmer for 1–2 minutes over a medium heat. Add asparagus and cook for a further 2 minutes before adding the tuna, pasta and rocket leaves. Squeeze over lemon juice and ¼ cup of pasta water. Stir to combine ingredients and cook for a further minute or so to heat and slightly wilt the rocket. If the pasta seems a little dry, add another ¼ cup of the pasta cooking water.

Serve with lots of freshly grated parmesan cheese and cracked black pepper.

tip Vegetarian versions of both recipes can be made by substituting tuna for extra parmesan. Together pasta and cheese is a complete protein source.

Fresh herbs and garlic give seafood a nutritional boost. Incorporate them into your seafood recipes whenever you can.

There are so many interesting varieties of pastas these days that cater for food allergies and healthy lifestyle choices. Check out your local health food store or larger supermarkets.

As you would expect, wholemeal varieties have more nutrients than white or refined pasta, so it is beneficial to try and include more of these into our diet. Select from wholemeal, spelt, rye, soya and buckwheat. You may find their flavours stronger than white pasta, but I think it only adds to a dish. They are also quite dense, so serving portions can be smaller. I have chosen buckwheat pasta for this recipe as it's excellent for digestion and varicose veins.

GOOD SOURCE OF: *omega 3, iodine, zinc, protein, carbohydrates, iron, calcium, fibre, vitamins A, C, D, K and B-group*

GOOD FOR MOTHER: *fatigue, constipation, strengthening blood vessels, iron absorption/anaemia, healthy blood and cells, hypertension, preparing uterus for birth, production of colostrum, lactation, reducing risk of osteoporosis and pre-term labour, skin elasticity*

GOOD FOR BABY: *brain and lung development, eyesight, weight gain, manufacture of baby's red blood cells, growth of hair, skin and body fat, strong healthy bones, teeth and nails*

177

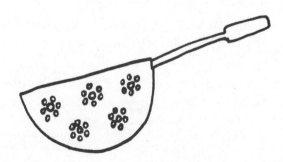

Chicken Fillets with Avocado and Almond Pesto

This pesto is from our beef pasta dish, but it is just too good to include in only one recipe. Make a batch of the pesto and have the beef dish one night and the chicken the next. Basil is known to tone the heart muscles and so is beneficial during the third trimester when your blood volume has doubled and the heart is working overtime to pump it around the body. Avocado and almonds are absolutely loaded with nutritional goodies to maintain your health while fuelling the rapid brain development of your baby.

2 chicken breast fillets

avocado and almond pesto (see recipe page 80)

big bowl of steamed vegetables

The chicken breasts can be grilled or cooked on the barbeque. Preheat your chosen cooking appliance.

Trim fat from chicken breasts and lightly baste with olive oil. Cook over a medium heat for approximately 5 minutes on each side, or until cooked all the way through.

While chicken is cooking, wash and prepare your vegetables. Place in a steamer and lightly steam until just tender.

Top chicken breast with a big dollop of pesto and serve with the steamed vegetables. The pesto is also fabulous stirred through the vegetables.

GOOD SOURCE OF: *protein, iron, vitamins B-group, C, E and K, selenium, phosphorus, potassium, zinc, essential fatty acids, calcium*

GOOD FOR MOTHER: *digestion, fatigue, anaemia, hypertension, reducing risk of pre-term labour and placental abruption, skin elasticity, healthy uterus for birth, lactation*

GOOD FOR BABY: *rapid brain development, production of baby's own blood supply, healthy skin, hair and eyes, strong bone and cell structure, muscle contractions, sexual development, functioning of nervous and immune systems*

Chicken Mango Salad

Yum yum! These ingredients could be combined simply for our tastebuds, but you cannot ignore the health benefits of this dish. Brimming with vitamins C and E, beta-carotene and other powerful antioxidants, this recipe will strengthen the immune system for excellent health, promote foetal growth and development and protect body cells and tissue against damage. It's hard to believe something that tastes so good can be so good for you.

2 sweet potatoes

1 bunch asparagus, or 150 g (5 oz) green beans

   cut into 3 cm lengths

1 avocado, sliced

1 mango, diced

½ red capsicum, thinly sliced

large handful of rocket, spinach, watercress

   or other dark mixed leaves

2 chicken breasts

cracked black pepper

pinch of cinnamon

dressing:

1 tbs flaxseed oil

1 tbs balsamic vinegar

cracked black pepper

179

Preheat oven to 180°C/350°F. Wash sweet potatoes thoroughly and cut into thin round slices.

Line a baking tray with baking paper, arrange sweet potato on the tray and bake for 30 minutes. If you are running short of time, boil the sweet potato for 5 minutes until just soft and then bake in the oven for 15 minutes until golden brown.

Trim asparagus by gently bending the base of each stem. The stalk will naturally snap at the point of tenderness. Discard woody ends and diagonally slice spears into 4 cm lengths. Steam the asparagus for 1–2 minutes, retaining a nice crunch. Remove from steamer and set aside to cool. Prepare avocado, mango, capsicum and rocket and place into a large salad bowl.

Trim chicken breasts of all visible white fat. Rinse with cold water and pat dry with a paper towel. Cut each fillet in half lengthways so you have four equally sized pieces. Season with black pepper and the cinnamon and use your fingers to rub the spices into the fillets.

Use a vegetable steamer and steam the chicken for 7–10 minutes, or until cooked through.

While the chicken is cooking, make the dressing. Whisk together the oil, vinegar and black pepper directly into a large salad bowl.

Remove chicken from steamer. Shred or finely slice and add to salad bowl with the dressing, asparagus and sweet potato. Mix well to combine ingredients.

GOOD SOURCE OF: *vitamins A, C, E, K and B-group, folate, antioxidants, protein, iron, potassium, fibre, essential fatty acids*

GOOD FOR MOTHER: *excellent health, dental problems, skin elasticity, hypertension, heartburn and reflux, fatigue, varicose veins, blood circulation, nourishing uterus and placenta, lactation, anaemia, iron absorption*

GOOD FOR BABY: *muscle contractions, development of healthy eyes, skin, hair, teeth and gums*

Rosemary, Lamb and Tomato Bake

This is another quick and easy meal that can be prepared in just 30 minutes. The combination of ingredients is fantastic for digestion, iron absorption and the production of haemoglobin. This is especially important during the third trimester as your baby begins to manufacture its own blood supply and lay its own iron stores down. It also reduces your risk of developing anaemia.

4 potatoes

1 red onion, quartered

1 punnet cherry tomatoes, halved

2 tbs fresh rosemary, chopped

400g (14 oz) trim lamb leg steaks

150g (5 oz) green beans or broccoli

dressing:

2 tbs olive oil

1 tbs balsamic vinegar

3 cloves garlic, crushed

cracked black pepper

Preheat oven to 160°C/320°F. Wash and cut potato into 3 cm pieces. Bring a medium saucepan of water to the boil. Add potatoes and cook for 5 minutes, or until just tender.

Prepare onion, tomatoes and rosemary and trim lamb of visible fat.

Whisk together dressing ingredients. Baste lamb with a little of the dressing.

Place empty baking dish in the oven for 5 minutes to heat.

Heat a non-stick frying pan and sear the lamb for 1 minute on each side. Take the pan off the heat and remove the baking dish from the oven. Place the lamb and all remaining ingredients into the dish and pour over the dressing. Use a large spoon to mix the ingredients together and coat with the dressing. Shake the pan to evenly distribute ingredients and return to the oven.

Bake for 15 minutes and serve with steamed broccoli or green beans.

181

GOOD SOURCE OF: *iron, protein, zinc, vitamins C, B6 and B12, folate, beta-carotene, fibre, potassium, phosphorus, selenium, antioxidants, carbohydrates*

GOOD FOR MOTHER: *anaemia, healthy blood, healthy heart, fatigue, digestion, circulation, hypertension, immunity, toning uterus*

GOOD FOR BABY: *providing building blocks for foetal growth, nervous and immune systems, nourishing bones, muscles, skin and organs, eyesight*

Mediterranean Lamb Pizzas

These mini pizzas are the perfect portion size for a shrinking stomach and provide close to all of the nutrients essential to the third trimester. Ingredients have been combined to maximise iron absorption, which is vital now as your baby starts to produce its own blood supply and your blood volume increases to its peak. The hummus is a high calcium source, but if your daily intake has not been met, add grated cheese to this recipe. Select from parmesan, cheddar or tasty.

½ punnet cherry tomatoes, halved, or 4 slow-roasted tomatoes

3 cloves garlic, crushed

juice of 1 lemon

1 tbs olive oil

3 sprigs fresh rosemary, leaves removed from stems and finely chopped

400 g (14 oz) trim lamb fillet, thinly sliced

½ cup button mushrooms, halved

4 wholemeal pita bases

hummus, homemade or bought

1 zucchini, thinly sliced

½ red capsicum, diced

2 marinated artichokes, drained and sliced

fresh rocket to serve

Preheat oven to 170°C/325°F. Prepare a baking tray and line it with baking paper.

Combine garlic, lemon juice, olive oil and 1 tablespoon of the rosemary. Add the lamb and mushrooms and marinate while preparing other ingredients.

If slow-roasting tomatoes, cut tomatoes lengthways, drizzle with balsamic vinegar and pepper and place in the oven for 10 minutes, or as long it is takes to prepare your pizzas for baking.

Spread pita bases generously with hummus. Arrange lamb slices and mushrooms on the hummus. Top with zucchini slices, capsicum and artichokes. Finally scatter with the tomatoes and remaining rosemary.

Bake for 10–15 minutes, or until the lamb is cooked through.

Serve with fresh rocket on top. Makes 4.

GOOD SOURCE OF: *iron, vitamins B6, B12 and C, folate, calcium, selenium, magnesium essential fatty acids*

GOOD FOR MOTHER: *fatigue, anaemia, digestion, circulation, constipation, hypertension, leg cramps, production of colostrum, reducing risk of osteoporosis, heart and kidney function*

GOOD FOR BABY: *supporting rapid foetal growth and developing blood supply, nerve and sexual development, growth of organs, hair, skin and fat, strong bones, teeth and nails*

Grilled Steak with Carrot and Walnut Salad

This dish serves up a good portion of your nutritional requirements for pregnancy and keeps you in excellent health. Its ingredients promote healthy red blood cell production for you and your baby, who is now producing his own supply. The salad is rich in vitamin C, making it great for iron absorption, immunity and healthy skin.

2 lean steaks (rump, New York or sirloin cuts)

marinade:

1 clove garlic

1 tsp cumin

juice of ½ large fresh orange

1 tbs olive oil

carrot and walnut salad:

2 carrots, grated

1 cup chopped fresh parsley

½ cup walnuts

½ cup currants

dressing:

2 tbs olive or grapeseed oil

1 tsp Dijon mustard

juice of ½ orange

cracked black pepper

184

Trim beef of visible fat. Mix marinade ingredients in a shallow bowl and rub into steaks. Cover and set aside in fridge for 30 minutes.

Grate carrots directly into large salad bowl. Add parsley, walnuts and currants. Combine dressing ingredients in a jar and shake vigorously. Dress salad and set aside while cooking meat. The dressing will plump the currants and infuse the flavours.

Barbeque or grill steak to your liking. Serve with carrot salad and steamed green beans.

GOOD SOURCE OF: *iron, protein, calcium, magnesium, omega 3, fibre, vitamins A, C and B12, folate*

GOOD FOR MOTHER: *anaemia, constipation, fatigue, immune system, skin elasticity, circulation, healthy skin, hair and bones for both mother and baby, lactation, preparing uterus for labour*

GOOD FOR BABY: *developing blood supply, organ growth, eyesight, nerve and muscle coordination, brain development, growth of hair, skin and body*

sesame Beef salad

This recipe is a shared experience. Ask your other half to barbeque or grill the steaks while you prepare the salad. It is a fabulous protein, iron and calcium source, providing the necessary building blocks for normal foetal growth. It also aims to build up your own stores, reducing the risk of anaemia and osteoporosis.

2 x 150 g (5 oz) lean beef steak

    (rump steak is a suitable cut)

1 bunch fresh asparagus

1 cucumber

2 shallots

1 carrot

2 large handfuls baby spinach leaves

⅓ cup coriander, chopped

1 tsp sesame seeds

sesame dressing:

1 tbs tahini

2–3 teaspoons lemon juice

1 small garlic clove, crushed

½ tsp cumin

⅓ cup plain, low-fat yoghurt

cracked black pepper

185

Preheat barbeque or grill.

To make the dressing, combine tahini and lemon juice and mix into a paste. Add garlic, cumin and the yoghurt and mix again to form a smooth texture. Season with black pepper.

Trim steaks of visible fat. Sear one side of the steaks on the preheated grill and cook for 3–4 minutes before turning. Cook for a further 3–4 minutes on the other side for a medium-cooked steak. For best results, only turn your steak once and always rest meat in a warm place for 5 minutes prior to serving. This allows cooking juices to settle.

Prepare salad ingredients. Bend to snap off tough asparagus ends and cut spears in half. Cook on the barbeque or grill for 3–4 minutes, or until just tender. Slice the cucumber and shallots in long diagonal lengths and use a vegetable peeler to prepare long, thin strips of carrot. Wash and pat dry the spinach leaves and coriander.

Roughly chop the coriander and place all ingredients into a large salad bowl, along with the sesame seeds. Feel free to toast these for a more intense flavour.

Cut steaks into 1 cm thick slices and add to the salad. Pour the dressing over the salad and toss to generously coat all salad ingredients.

GOOD SOURCE OF: *iron, protein, vitamins A, C, E, K, B1, B6 and B12, folate, fibre, phosphorus, potassium, magnesium, essential fatty acids, calcium, antioxidants*

GOOD FOR MOTHER: *fatigue, anaemia, iron absorption, skin elasticity, immunity, strengthening blood vessels, nourishing placenta, toning uterus, protecting cells from damage, lactation, leg cramps*

GOOD FOR BABY: *strong bones, nervous system, growth of healthy skin, hair and eyes, teeth and nails*

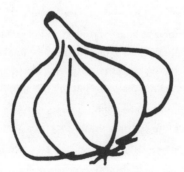

PORK with RED Cabbage SaLaD

This is a refreshing and crunchy salad that helps to prevent most of the common complaints of the third trimester. The rainbow of colours in this salad indicates that it contains a good variety of essential nutrients. Pork is rich in thiamine, imperative for maternal and foetal growth. It breaks down carbohydrates to energy for both mother and baby. This is also a great dish to combat anaemia as red cabbage is rich in chlorophyll, which is known to restore red blood cells to normal levels.

2 cups red cabbage, finely sliced

1 medium carrot, grated

4 leaves of silverbeet or half a bunch
   of English spinach

2 stalks celery, sliced

½ cup currants

½ cup sesame seeds

1 x 200g (7 oz) pork fillet or butterfly steaks

dressing:

½ cup (125 ml/4 fl oz) grape seed
   or olive oil

½ cup (125 ml/4 fl oz) orange juice

1 tsp Dijon mustard

cracked black pepper

Heat barbeque plate or grill.

Place all dressing ingredients in a jar and shake to combine.

Toss all remaining ingredients, except for the pork, into a salad bowl. Add salad dressing.

Grill or barbeque pork fillet, ensuring fillet is cooked through. Cut pork into 2 cm thick slices and arrange on serving plates. Serve with red cabbage salad.

GOOD SOURCE OF: *protein, vitamins C, B5 and B12, folate, omega 3, calcium, magnesium, beta-carotene, fibre, essential fatty acids*

GOOD FOR MOTHER: *healthy blood/anaemia, fatigue, bleeding gums, hypertension, digestion, diabetes, constipation, fluid retention, stretch marks, varicose veins, boosting immune system*

GOOD FOR BABY: *production of baby's red blood cells, healthy lungs, eyesight, strong teeth and bones*

Roast Vegetable and Soft Egg Salad

Baking is a healthy and nutritional way of cooking vegetables. I highly recommend you use leeks and mushrooms in this dish. They go very well with eggs and release sweet-tasting juices during cooking that do wonders for this dish. They also reduce the amount of oil needed, so you may find the need for an extra tablespoon if not using either of these vegetables. Select from at least five of the vegetables listed.

sweet potato, parsnip, carrot, red capsicum, mushrooms, leeks, red onion, zucchini, tomato (in equal quantities, or according to taste)

1 tbs olive oil

3 garlic cloves

½ cup fresh parsley or basil, chopped

cracked black pepper

white wine vinegar

2 eggs, preferably biodynamic

generous handful of baby spinach leaves

Preheat oven to 180°C/350°F on fan-forced setting.

Cut all vegetables, except for mushrooms and tomatoes, into 2–3cm lengths.

Warm a baking tray in the oven.

Steam the sweet potato, parsnip and carrots for 4–5 minutes.

Remove the baking dish from oven and add the oil. Swirl or baste to coat the base of the pan. Add all vegetables except the spinach leaves, garlic and parsley and shake the pan to coat the veges with the oil.

Peel the garlic cloves and gently press down on the whole clove with a knife and the heel of your palm to slightly split the clove open. Add the garlic and herbs and season with black pepper. Shake the pan again and bake for 20 minutes, turning vegetables once or twice to blend the flavours. The cooking aroma of this dish is simply heavenly.

Test vegetables are cooked by inserting a fork into the starchy vegetables. Turn the oven off but leave the vegetables in the oven while you poach the eggs.

Fill a deep frying pan with water and add 2 tablespoons white wine vinegar. Bring to a gentle simmer and poach eggs for 4–5 minutes to ensure egg yolks are cooked. Remove with a slotted spoon and drain on a paper towel.

Remove vegetables from the oven and mix through the spinach leaves. Divide between two serving plates and gently place a poached egg on each. Season to taste with black pepper. Serves 2.

tip *Poached eggs can be replaced with boiled eggs. Always ensure your eggs are fully cooked as expecting mothers should not eat runny yolks*

GOOD SOURCE OF: *protein, complex carbohydrates, zinc, iodine, omega 3, vitamins A, D and B-group, selenium, potassium*

GOOD FOR MOTHER: *healthy blood and uterus, fluid retention, hypertension, circulation, skin elasticity*

GOOD FOR BABY: *fuelling growth and development, building muscles, bones, skin and organs, strong cell structure, brain development*

Quinoa Capsicum Treats

Quinoa is a high-quality protein grain. In fact, it contains more protein than any other grain and provides all of the essential amino acids normally only found in animal products. Unlike animal products, quinoa contains no saturated fat and is very easy to digest. While it is a fantastic food choice for vegetarians, I urge everyone to try this wonderful grain. It is gluten free and has a low GI rating for sustained energy and to regulate blood sugar levels. It is also a very light grain and therefore perfect for the third trimester.

Quinoa is available from health food stores and can be used in a variety of dishes as you would rice, pasta or couscous. It can even be stewed with prunes, pears or apricots and served with nuts and yoghurt for an interesting alternative to porridge.

In this recipe I use quinoa as a savoury filling for capsicums. I have offered two recipes for a bit of variation as I hope quinoa becomes a regular grain in your diet.

GOOD SOURCE OF: *protein, vitamins C, B6, B12 and D, beta-carotene, omega 3, essential fatty acids, calcium, potassium*

GOOD FOR MOTHER: *vegetarian and gluten-free diets, fertility, diabetes, digestion, fatigue, skin elasticity, circulation, immunity, constipation, anaemia, healthy blood and heart, hypertension, uterus and muscle strength*

GOOD FOR BABY: *brain development, function of nervous and immune systems, building muscles, bones, skin and organs, production of baby's own blood supply and iron stores*

Preparing Quinoa and Capsicums

½ cup quinoa

2 cups (500 ml/16 fl oz) water

2 capsicums

Preheat oven to 170°C/325°F.

Cook the quinoa in the water in a covered saucepan for 10–15 minutes, or until all water has been absorbed and grain is light and fluffy. Slice the capsicums in half lengthways to get two boat-like halves. Remove seeds and pith.

Cheese, Mushroom and Quinoa Capsicum Treats

2 tsp olive oil

100g (3½ oz) mushrooms

1 clove garlic, crushed

1 shallot, diced

cracked black pepper

splash of balsamic vinegar (optional)

3 tbs grated hard cheese

½ cup almonds

½ cup currants

½ cup parsley

Prepare quinoa and capsicums as above.

Heat the olive oil in a small pan, add the mushrooms, garlic and shallots and stir-fry for 3–4 minutes until mushrooms soften. Season with pepper and balsamic vinegar.

Remove quinoa from heat and add the mushroom mixture to the saucepan with 2 tablespoons of the cheese. Mix through and then add all remaining ingredients.

Place capsicums in a baking tray and spoon in the quinoa mixture. Pack the mixture firmly into the capsicums and top with remaining cheese.

Bake for 15–20 minutes, by which time the capsicums with be slightly softened.

Spiced Quinoa And Avocado Capsicum Treats

½ avocado, diced

1 tbs sesame seeds

½ cup almonds

½ cup currants

½ cup parsley

1 tomato, diced

2 shallots, diced

10 mint leaves

½ tsp fennel seeds

pinch ground cumin

2 tsp balsamic vinegar

cracked black pepper

wheatgerm

Preheat oven to 170°C/325°F.

Prepare quinoa and capsicums as above.

Remove quinoa from heat and, while warm, add the avocado to the pan. Stir through and then add all remaining ingredients. Season with black pepper.

Place capsicums in a baking tray and spoon in the quinoa mixture. Firmly pack the mixture in and sprinkle with wheatgerm. Bake for 15–20 minutes.

tip *Both fillings can be eaten as meals on their own, or as a side dish with any meat. The spiced avocado, in particular, is a perfect work lunch option.*

Pears, Cheese and Oatmeal Biscuits

Cheese lovers do have to make some sacrifices during pregnancy. Sadly, there are no substitutes for soft, smelly cheeses, so let's make the most of the fabulous hard cheeses available. Choose from aged parmesan, tasty and cheddar cheeses, or a mild edam cheese. These four varieties are your best nutritional choices during pregnancy. Team them with some delicious oatmeal biscuits and a fresh, crisp pear and you might just consider it the next best thing.

> 4 oatmeal or wheatmeal biscuits
>
> 1 firm but ripe pear (Beurre bosc goes well)
>
> 60 g (2½ oz) hard cheese (select from parmesan, tasty, cheddar or edam)

Top an oatmeal biscuit with thin slices of pear and thick slices of cheese.

Despite its goodness, cheese is high in saturated fat, so do eat in moderation!

193

GOOD SOURCE OF: *protein, calcium, magnesium, vitamins A, D, K and B-group, zinc*

GOOD FOR MOTHER: *digestion, cleansing, fatigue, reducing risk of osteoporosis, cell growth, leg cramps, hypertension, normal kidney function*

GOOD FOR BABY: *strong bones and teeth, healthy skin and eyes, good vision, bone and body-building, resistance against infection, nervous system*

Chocolate and Beetroot Cake

This wheat-free chocolate cake is oozing with goodness. Beetroot and chocolate may sound like a strange combination, but the flavours are simply fabulous together. They are also excellent tonics for promoting healthy blood. This is very beneficial during the third trimester as your blood volume doubles in quantity. This cake is wonderful served straight from the oven as a winter dessert. Serve with vanilla or plain yoghurt.

1 medium raw beetroot, to yield 1 cup grated

zest and juice of 2 large oranges, to yield 1 cup/250 ml/8 fl oz orange juice

2 tbs honey

3 eggs

⅓ cup cocoa powder

3 tsp baking powder

2 tsp cinnamon

2 tbs brown rice flour

200 g (7 oz) almond meal

yoghurt to serve

194

Preheat oven to 170°C/325°F. Line a 22 cm round cake tin with baking paper.

Peel beetroot and grate to yield 1 cup. Zest oranges and add to beetroot.

Combine honey and orange juice and stir to dissolve.

Beat the eggs, then add orange juice mixture and blend until nice and creamy. Sift cocoa and baking powder, cinnamon and brown rice flour. Add to egg mixture and process until combined.

Use a large metal spoon and gently fold through the almond meal, grated beetroot and orange zest until just combined. Pour mixture into prepared cake tin. Bake for 30 minutes, or until cooked. Check by inserting a skewer into the centre of the cake. If the skewer comes out clean, the cake is cooked; if there is mixture on the end, cook for a further 5 minutes.

Either serve warm with your favourite yoghurt or cool the cake in the pan before turning on to a cake rack to cool completely. Store in an airtight container in a cool place for 3–4 days. In the warmer weather, this is best kept in the fridge for freshness.

GOOD SOURCE OF: *protein, iron, calcium, magnesium, potassium, phosphorus, vitamins E and B-group, essential fatty acids, antioxidants*

GOOD FOR MOTHER: *healthy blood/anaemia, fatigue, hypertension, gluten-free diets, skin elasticity/stretch marks, digestion, toning uterus for labour, reducing damage to tissue and arteries, calcium absorption, leg cramps, liver and kidneys*

GOOD FOR BABY: *healthy brain and heart, muscle contractions, nerve function, strong bones, organ growth, baby's blood supply*

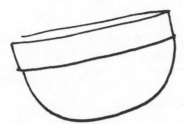

Bananas in Pyjamas

Bananas are packed with nourishment, especially potassium, essential to the functioning of every single cell in the body, and magnesium, which helps retain calcium in the bones. Baked bananas are delicious wrapped up in light, crispy filo.

juice of 1 orange

½ tsp mixed spice

1 tsp honey

2 bananas, peeled

6 filo sheets

2 tbs olive oil

1 tbs wheatgerm

Preheat oven to 180°C/350°F. Line a baking tray with baking paper.

Combine orange juice, spice and honey in a shallow bowl and coat bananas.

Prepare a clean, flat surface (either a large chopping board or bench top) and lay out one sheet of filo pastry, brush with oil and sprinkle with a little wheatgerm. Repeat with the remaining sheets of filo, but do not baste the top of the final sheet.

Cut filo sheets in half to form two even squares. Place the banana in the middle of the pastry square on the diagonal. Pour a little of the orange juice marinade over the banana, reserving some to baste the finished parcels. Brush the pastry edges with water. Fold the corner of pastry over the banana to form a triangle—the corner should come about 2–3 cm short of the opposite corner. Fold over the two end corners and firmly press the edges into the pastry and brush again with water to seal the edges. Now roll the pastry and banana towards the furthest corner to form a neat parcel. Repeat procedure and then baste the top of each parcel with remaining orange juice.

Transfer to prepared baking tray and cook for 20 minutes, or until pastry is golden brown. Serve warm with your favourite yoghurt. Makes 2.

GOOD SOURCE OF: *potassium, magnesium, folate, vitamins B6 and B12, calcium*

GOOD FOR MOTHER: *digestion, fatigue, eliminating waste, hypertension, leg cramps, calcium absorption*

GOOD FOR BABY: *development of brain and nervous system, healthy body cells, hardening of bones*

Tofu Berry Cream

Tofu is an excellent and complete source of protein, calcium and dietary fibre. This recipe is the perfect introduction to tofu if you are not familiar with its taste and texture. When blended with frozen fruit it produces a thick creamy texture and a healthy non-dairy substitute for ice-cream. It is light, refreshing and easy to digest. Perfect for the third trimester and lactation. You do have to pre-plan and freeze the banana and berries overnight.

1 frozen banana

1 cup frozen blueberries/mixed berries

1 cup silken tofu

½ cup (125 ml/4 fl oz) fresh orange juice

½ tsp vanilla extract

Peel one banana, wrap in cling wrap and freeze overnight. Freeze 1 cup of berries. Place all ingredients in blender and process until thick and creamy. Serve immediately.

197

GOOD SOURCE OF: *protein, calcium, magnesium, potassium, vitamins C and B-group, fibre, antioxidants*

GOOD FOR MOTHER: *calcium stores, constipation, skin elasticity, dental problems, fatigue, anaemia, immune system, maintaining health of all major organs, breasts and uterus*

GOOD FOR BABY: *development of baby's lungs, circulatory systems and healthy blood supply, strong teeth, nails and bones, development of muscles, skin and organs, building muscle strength*

Grilled figs with cinnamon

This simple dish makes the most of seasonal produce. Figs are only available for a few precious months of the year, so enjoy them while you can. Fresh figs are bursting with nutrition and are an excellent source of dietary fibre, so they will come in handy for many during the last phase of pregnancy. Serve figs with your favourite yoghurt for a low-fat dessert rich in protein, calcium and containing absolutely no sugar.

3–4 fresh figs

1 tsp cinnamon

low-fat yoghurt to serve, *vanilla or raspberry flavours go very well*

Preheat grill to a medium heat. Slice figs in half and lightly sprinkle with cinnamon. Place under the grill for 10 minutes so the cinnamon dissolves into the figs. Serve with a generous dollop of yoghurt.

198

tip *Slivered almonds are also a delightful addition. Sprinkle over figs and grill.*

GOOD SOURCE OF: *fibre, potassium, calcium, magnesium, protein, vitamins A, B12 and D*

GOOD FOR MOTHER: *constipation, healthy digestive tract, regulating blood sugar levels, fluid retention*

GOOD FOR BABY: *muscle contractions, nerve transmission, eyesight, immunity*

❋ General Recipes for Pregnancy

Snacks

Sides

Ways with Bread

Drinks

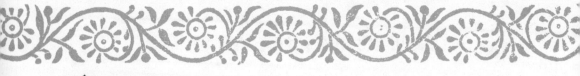

❀ Snacks

Snacks are an essential component of the pregnancy diet. You should always carry a supply in your bag, and stock up at work. They are an instant energy source, provide bonus nutrients and control blood sugar levels and fatigue. A combination of carbohydrate and protein is recommended for snacking. Try to eat every 2 to 3 hours, even if it is just a banana or a fresh fruit smoothie.

Some fabulous snack recipes follow and most can be pre-made and frozen so that healthy options are always on hand when hunger strikes. Some of these snack recipes are particularly helpful to certain trimesters, but generally they can be enjoyed throughout your entire pregnancy. Snacks are also beneficial during lactation. You will find an extensive section on suggested sandwich fillings and toast toppings that work well between meals.

Some of the best snacks require minimal or no cooking. You can't go wrong with any of the following healthy choices:

- nuts and seeds—almonds, peanuts, brazil nuts, walnuts, sunflower seeds, pepitas and sesame seeds
- dried fruit—mix in with your nuts, or enjoy on their own; dried apricots, sultanas and prunes are good low GI choices and high in fibre
- hard cheese—slice or cube cheddar or edam cheese or grab a cheese stick for an instant calcium hit; team with sesame or wholegrain crackers or make a cheese sandwich on wholegrain bread for a more substantial snack
- roasted chickpeas—calcium and protein rich and available from health food stores
- canned tuna/salmon slices—protein and omega 3 rich
- boiled eggs—nature's very own multi-vitamin capsule
- raw vegetables with hummus—calcium, protein and vitamin rich
- tub of low-fat yoghurt—calcium rich and a healthy sweet fix
- milkshakes and smoothies—homemade or purchased; add a tablespoon of wheatgerm
- healthy muffins—homemade, or locate a store that sells healthy ones
- stewed fruit—select from pears, peaches, plums, apricots and apples.

Nourishing Nut and Seed Mix

Nuts are an important food source during pregnancy. This combination of nuts and seeds boasts most of the essential nutrients and should be eaten throughout your pregnancy. It's the perfect on-the-go snack, or can be added to almost any recipe. Sprinkle over salads, steamed veges, sandwich fillings and cereals. Nuts are nourishing but they are also high in fat, so dietitians recommend eating only a third of a cup per day.

Cooking brings out the flavour in seeds and nuts. You can either oven roast or dry fry in a non-stick frying pan. Make up a large batch and store in the fridge for freshness.

1 cup each of pepitas, almonds, sunflower seeds and sesame seeds

To Roast: Preheat oven to 160°C/320°F. Place a sheet of baking paper on a large roasting tray. Spread nuts on to the paper evenly and place in the middle shelf of the oven. Check after 5 minutes and gently shake nuts. Check again at 10 minutes. Nuts and seeds can burn easily so cook on low temperatures and keep an eye on them during cooking. Remove when just golden brown, which usually takes about 10 minutes.

Slide the baking paper and nuts on to a cake cooling rack and cool completely. It is important to remove the nuts/seeds from the hot tray as the heat can continue to cook (and burn) them.

To Dry Fry: Heat a heavy-based, non-stick frying pan over a low-medium heat. Add nut and seed mixture and gently shake the pan to distribute evenly. Cook for 2–3 minutes, or until golden brown, shaking mixture occasionally to prevent burning. If the nuts or seeds begin to 'pop' remove from heat immediately.

Slide nuts on to a sheet of baking paper positioned on a cake cooling rack to cool.

tip *Warm nuts do loose their crunch, but this will return once cooled. After cooking, cool completely before storing. To ensure freshness store in the refrigerator in an airtight container or glass jar. Nuts do go stale and some can turn rancid, particularly walnuts.*

GOOD SOURCE OF: *protein, essential fatty acids, calcium, magnesium, zinc, potassium, fibre*

GOOD FOR MOTHER: *fertility, fatigue, hypertension, leg cramps, skin elasticity, circulation, lactation, healthy heart, liver and kidneys, reducing risk of pre-term labour*

GOOD FOR BABY: *muscle contractions, development of brain and nervous system, fuelling foetal growth*

Tamari Roasted Almonds

Almonds are packed with nutrients and are a perfect high-protein snack. Tamari is a wheat-free soy sauce and gives the almonds a scrumptious flavour. Serve warm or cold. Eat in moderation . . . if you can.

150 g (5 oz) natural almonds

1 tbs salt-reduced tamari (wheat-free soy sauce)

Preheat oven to 160°C/320°F.

Pour nuts into a shallow baking tray or loaf tin. Roast for 5 minutes. Remove from the oven and drizzle over the tamari. Shake pan to coat the almonds. Return to the oven and roast for a further 5 minutes, shaking the pan frequently to avoid sticking or burning. Remove from the oven and pour the nuts on to a flat plate to cool. Serve warm or cool completely before storing in an airtight container.

GOOD SOURCE OF: *protein, calcium, potassium, magnesium, zinc, riboflavin, essential fatty acids*

GOOD FOR MOTHER: *preconception, fertility, healthy skin, skin elasticity, hormone production, immune and nervous systems, digestion, reducing risk of pre-term labour*

GOOD FOR BABY: *brain development, reproduction and growth, strong cell structure, strong teeth and bones*

Hummus

Hummus is a perfect example of combining vegetables (chickpeas and sesame seeds) to achieve a complete protein source. My twist on traditional hummus is the addition of yoghurt for added calcium. Hummus is very versatile. Spread it on toast, sandwiches and pizza bases, use as a healthy dip with vitamin C-rich raw vegetables, or over grilled chicken or lamb.

I highly recommend you have a fresh batch of hummus on hand throughout your entire pregnancy.

> 2 cups canned chickpeas
>
> ½ cup yoghurt, or silken tofu
>
> 2 tbs tahini
>
> 2 tbs fresh lemon juice
>
> ⅛ tsp ground cumin
>
> 1 clove garlic, crushed (optional)
>
> cracked black pepper
>
> 1 tsp olive oil

Place chickpeas and yoghurt into a food processor and blend until just combined. Add tahini, lemon juice, cumin, garlic and black pepper and blend again to form a smooth paste. Drizzle in the olive oil and process for 30 seconds.

tip *Store in an airtight container in the refrigerator. Hummus keeps for 4–5 days and is also suitable for freezing. To increase the quantity, simply double all ingredients with ¼ teaspoon of cumin.*

GOOD SOURCE OF: *protein, calcium, iron, folate, vitamin B12, fibre, magnesium, potassium*

GOOD FOR MOTHER: *vegetarians, fatigue, constipation, diabetes, digestion, skin elasticity/stretch marks, leg cramps, manufacture of red blood cells and body cells, healthy kidneys, reducing risk of osteoporosis, anaemia and spina bifida*

GOOD FOR BABY: *development of brain, spine, organs and nervous system, strong bones, teeth and nails, healthy skin and eyes, regulating heartbeat*

Tasty Tuna Patties

These tasty little patties proved to be the most popular snack with my recipe testers. They are the perfect portable meal or snack and a great portion size for later in the third trimester, when smaller meals are called for. They can also be made in batches and frozen for individual use, ideal for the first few months of motherhood. Two of our pregnancy superfoods—tuna and chickpeas—are the main ingredients in this recipe, making it a highly nutritious choice.

200 g dried or 1 cup canned chickpeas

1 medium-sized sweet potato

1 brown onion

½ red capsicum

1 cup parsley or coriander

1 x 425 g (4½ oz) can tuna in olive oil

juice of one lemon

2 tbs milk

1 tsp cumin

1 egg, lightly whisked

2 tbs wheatgerm

⅓ cup plain flour

1 extra egg to coat patties for baking

Cook chickpeas or thoroughly rinse canned chickpeas through a strainer at least three times to remove salt preservatives.

Wash and roughly chop the sweet potato. Bring a medium saucepan of water to the boil and cook sweet potato for 10–15 minutes, or until soft.

Preheat oven to 180°C/350°F and line a baking tray with baking paper.

Finely dice the onion and capsicum and finely chop the herbs. Drain the tuna of the canned oil and flake into small pieces. Drizzle tuna with lemon juice.

Strain sweet potato and transfer to a large mixing bowl, along with the chickpeas. Add the milk, cumin and some black pepper and mash. Add the mash to the tuna mixture, together with the whisked egg and wheatgerm. Mix ingredients together (best done with hands).

Pour flour on to a clean surface or large chopping board and whisk the extra egg in a bowl. Form dessertspoonfuls of the mixture into patties. Lightly roll the patties in the flour and dip into the egg. Place on prepared baking tin and repeat until all the mixture has been used. It will make about 12 patties. Place into the oven and bake for 25 minutes, or until golden brown.

These tuna patties can be served with a dollop of yoghurt and a fresh salad on the side, or as a burger. Place the patty on a wholegrain roll spread with light cream cheese or yoghurt and top with dark salad leaves and some slices of fresh tomato and cucumber.

GOOD SOURCE OF: *omega 3, fibre, iron, iodine, protein, calcium, zinc, magnesium, vitamins C and B-group*

GOOD FOR MOTHER: *fatigue, diabetes, constipation, production of collagen/skin elasticity, healthy blood, heart and kidneys, leg cramps, reproduction, cell growth, muscle contractions*

GOOD FOR BABY: *development of brain, eyes, organs, skeleton, nervous and circulatory systems, strong bones and teeth*

205

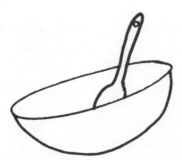

The Easiest Rice Paper Rolls

I love rice papers rolls. They are so cleansing and during pregnancy they are a wonderful way to eat lots of raw, fresh vegetables. They might also assist in aversions to protein as the protein source is wrapped up in an abundance of fragrant and tasty vegetables. They are a light yet substantial snack or perfect smaller meal portion for later in the third trimester.

Rice paper rolls are really an Asian version of the sandwich wrap. Instead of wheat-based flat bread we have a light, rice-based alternative. Traditional rice paper rolls involve the time-consuming, paper-thin slicing of ingredients. My version is to make a big salad and roll up small portions in the rice paper. It is not nearly as fiddly and once you have the hang of the rolling technique, preparation is fun and fast.

I have listed my favourite salad filling ingredients, but this can vary according to taste as long as you include a wide variety of fresh crunchy veges. The herbs, however, are imperative to the traditional Asian flavour. I don't use vermicelli in my rolls as I would rather fill them up with more vegetables, but I do love adding thin slices of mango for an unexpected twist and a great boost of vitamin C.

For nutritional purposes, always include a protein source. Choose from tofu, shredded chicken breast, thinly sliced wok-seared beef, pork, cooked prawns or even canned salmon or tuna.

1 cucumber, finely diced

6 snow peas or 1 stick celery, finely diced

½ red capsicum, finely diced

2 shallots, finely diced

½ medium carrot, grated

½ mango, thinly sliced or ½ avocado, thinly sliced

1 cup baby spinach leaves or lettuce leaves finely shredded

½ cup fresh coriander leaves, chopped

½ cup fresh mint leaves, shredded

150–200 g (5–7 oz) protein, as suggested above

10–12 large rice paper wrappers

hoi-sin dipping sauce:

2 tbs hoi-sin sauce

3 tsp rice wine vinegar

chilli and lime dipping sauce:

2 tbs sweet chilli sauce

1 tbs lime juice

1 tsp fresh chives

Prepare all salad ingredients and combine in a large bowl. Canned fish, shredded chicken or thinly sliced beef could also now be added to the salad. Cooked prawns or sliced tofu can be added separately to each individual roll.

To prepare the rolls you will need a large bowl a little wider than your rice paper sheet. You will also need a plastic chopping board or damp, clean tea towel spread over your work surface in order to assemble the rolls. You will need another damp tea towel or paper towel to cover the prepared rolls to prevent them from drying out.

Fill the bowl with lukewarm water. Gently submerge a rice paper sheet in the water for about 30 seconds or until it is *just* soft and pliable (it will continue to soften as you roll). If you soak the paper for too long it will tear when you roll. Gently remove the rice paper and lay it on your working surface.

Place a heaped dessertspoon size of the salad mixture about a third of the way from the edge closest to you. Leave approximately 2 cm clear on each side of the rice paper to fold over. Fold the edge closest to you up and over the mixture. Firmly fold the two sides in and roll away from you. Lightly press the edge to secure, and place edge-side down on your prepared plate, covering with the edges of the tea towel to keep moist. Repeat with the remaining wrappers and filling.

Serve with your chosen dipping sauce. Makes 10–12.

207

tip *Rice paper rolls are best eaten fresh on the day of preparation. Wrap in a damp paper towel and store in an airtight container for a few hours.*

GOOD SOURCE OF: *protein, iron, selenium, calcium, vitamins A, C and B-group, folate*

GOOD FOR MOTHER: *digestion, fatigue, circulation, fluid retention, healthy skin, eyes, teeth and gums, immune system, food aversions, fertility, iron absorption, dental problems, good health*

GOOD FOR BABY: *development of spine and neural tube, reducing risk of birth defects, formation of skin, hair, ears and external structures, cell growth*

The Healthiest Spring Rolls

You will never want to eat deep-fried spring rolls after you make and taste this version thanks to The Golden Door Health Retreat. They are easy to prepare and so unbelievably healthy. Impress guests with these starters at your next dinner, or simply treat yourself as a snack or light meal. All the goodness of salmon and asparagus is bundled up with finely shredded cabbage. Cabbage is rich in vitamins C and A, which strengthen the immune system, promote excellent eyesight and maximise iron absorption.

300g (11 oz) salmon fillets

10 sheets (22 x 23 cm) spring roll pastry wrappers

½ small Chinese cabbage, shredded

2 bunches fresh asparagus spears

½ bunch fresh coriander leaves

30 g (1¼ oz) pickled ginger, sliced

1 egg white, to glaze

Preheat oven to 200°C. Slice the salmon fillets into ten 9 x 2 cm lengths.

Place one sheet of pastry on a clean, dry, flat surface. Place a small pile of cabbage on the pastry—you will need enough to form an effective layer between the pastry and the remaining filling. Place a piece of salmon on top, then an asparagus spear, some fresh coriander leaves and pickled ginger.

Fold the pastry from the bottom end over the filling and continue rolling until halfway up the pastry sheet. Now fold the left side of the pastry over, then fold the right side over. Continue rolling until pastry is finished and the roll is sealed. Repeat with remaining pastry and filling.

Place spring rolls seam-side down on a baking tray and lightly brush with egg white. Bake for 15 minutes, or until golden brown. Either serve whole or cut in half diagonally. They are tasty on their own or served with a small bowl of hoi-sin dipping sauce (see Rice Paper Rolls).

Makes 10. Best eaten on the day of preparation.

Spring roll wrappers are available in the freezer section of most supermarkets. Pickled ginger is available in some supermarkets, otherwise Asian supermarkets or sushi outlets sell small portions for next to nothing. Copyright, accreditation and thanks to The Golden Door, Australia.

GOOD SOURCE OF: *protein, iron, iodine, zinc, omega 3, selenium, potassium, vitamins A, C, E, K and B-group including folate*

GOOD FOR MOTHER: *high blood pressure, constipation, healthy blood, anaemia, blood sugar levels, fatigue, diabetes, circulation, nausea, immunity, extra blood supply, skin elasticity, toning uterus, tissue healing, fluid retention, nourishing placenta*

GOOD FOR BABY: *development of brain, eyes, immune and central nervous systems, fuelling foetal growth, healthy teeth and gums, strong bones, rapidly developing body cells and red blood cells*

Tuna, Leek and Mushroom sauté

Despite all your good intentions, there will be times when you don't want to cook. You've had a busy day, there's nothing in the fridge and you're exhausted. Ironically, these are the days you need a nourishing meal the most, to refuel and recharge. This recipe was created after one of those days. Using three basic ingredients, I came up with a concoction that was tasty, healthy and on the table in just ten minutes.

Canned tuna should be a pantry staple. It is a great source of omega 3, iodine and protein for brain function and overall excellent wellbeing.

150 g (5 oz) mushrooms, halved

1 small leek

1 small garlic clove, crushed

110 g (4 oz) can tuna in springwater

½ tsp dried thyme

cracked black pepper

2 slices wholegrain toast

Heat 2 teaspoon olive oil in a non-stick frying pan. Add mushrooms, leek and garlic and cook for 5–8 minutes, until leeks are soft. Stir through tuna, season with thyme and pepper and cook for another 1–2 minutes to warm tuna through.

Serve on wholegrain or cape seed toast.

GOOD SOURCE OF: *omega 3, iodine, iron, protein, potassium, phosphorus, selenium, vitamins D, E and B-group*

GOOD FOR MOTHER: *fertility, fatigue, fluid retention, hypertension, diabetes, skin elasticity, healthy blood and heart, normal blood clotting, production of haemoglobin and genetic material*

GOOD FOR BABY: *development of brain, eyes, muscles, skin, organs, immune and central nervous systems*

Chocolate Spiced Muffins

Here is a chocolate treat that is low in fat and guilt-free. In fact, it's actually good for you. Dried fruit and mixed spice are used to naturally sweeten the muffins and I have used buckwheat flour for its excellent nutritional and health properties. It is very friendly to the digestive tract, controls high blood pressure and is known to help prevent the onset of varicose veins. Cocoa, of course, is a useful source of iron, so please . . . enjoy!

⅔ cup dates

⅔ cup pitted prunes

1 cup water

½ tsp bicarbonate of soda

1 cup (250 ml/8 fl oz) buttermilk

½ cup (125ml/4 fl oz) oil

1½ cups self-raising wholemeal flour

½ cup buckwheat flour

4 tsp mixed spice

½ cup cocoa

1 tsp baking powder

1 tbs LSA

1 egg

211

Preheat oven to 180°C/350°F. Grease a 12 cup muffin tin.

Roughly chop dried fruit, removing all seeds. Place the dried fruit and water into a small saucepan. Bring to the boil, cover and reduce to simmer for 2 minutes. Add the bicarbonate of soda and simmer for a further 30 seconds. The mixture will foam when the soda is added. Turn off heat and add the milk and oil to the saucepan. Combine and let mixture cool slightly.

Sift flours, mixed spice, cocoa and baking powder into a large mixing bowl. Tip remaining husk flakes in the sifter into the bowl, together with the linseed, sunflower and almond meal.

Use a large metal spoon and fold a few times to combine the dry ingredients. Lightly beat the eggs in a separate bowl.

Create a well in the centre of the dry ingredients and pour in the fruit mixture. Use a large metal spoon to gently fold through the wet ingredients until just combined. Finally, add the eggs and again fold through until just combined. Spoon the mixture evenly into the muffin cases.

Bake for 15 minutes, checking by inserting a skewer into the centre of the muffin. If the skewer comes out clean the muffins are ready; if not, allow them to cook for a further 5 minutes.

Let the muffins cool a little in the tin before turning them on to a cake rack to cool completely.

Muffins will keep in an airtight container for 3–4 days. They are also suitable to freeze. Makes 12.

tip *If you do not have buckwheat flour, simply substitute with ¼ cup self-raising wholemeal flour. For those at high risk of developing gestational diabetes, substitute the dates for extra prunes for a lower GI rated recipe.*

GOOD SOURCE OF: *calcium, iron, protein, fibre, vitamins A, E and B-group, potassium, magnesium*

GOOD FOR MOTHER: *fatigue, digestion, varicose veins, circulation, constipation, energy source, healthy liver, supporting increased blood supply, skin and eyes*

GOOD FOR BABY: *strong bones, teeth and nails, promoting overall foetal growth, muscle/brain coordination*

pear, Raspberry and oat Muffins

Low in fat, high in fibre and packed with goodness. This is a delicious muffin to have for breakfast, as a snack or to serve with yoghurt as a dessert. The gorgeous blend of the raspberries, pear and rosewater gives the muffins a subtle, feminine flavour, making them perfect to serve at the baby shower.

1½ cups wholemeal flour

2 tsp baking powder

1 cup oats

½ cup oat bran

2 eggs, beaten

1 cup plain low-fat yoghurt

1 heaped tbs honey

¼ cup (60 ml/2 fl oz) olive oil

1 tsp rosewater (optional)

2 ripe pears, grated (skin on if organic)

½ cup raspberries (if frozen, thawed and drained)

213

Preheat oven to 180°C/350°F. Line each 12 cups of a muffin tin with a square sheet of baking paper to form a case approximately 2 cm higher than the tray.

Sift flour and baking soda into a large mixing bowl. Tip the husk flakes from the sifted flour into the bowl. Add oats and oat bran and gently combine by folding over with a large metal spoon.

Beat eggs in a medium-sized mixing bowl. Add yoghurt, honey, oil and rosewater and whisk together with a fork. Gently fold through grated pears and raspberries.

Make a well in the centre of the dry ingredients and add egg mixture. Fold through, from the inside out, until just combined. Do not over-mix. Spoon into cases.

Bake for 20–25 minutes, until golden and spongy to the touch. Insert a skewer into the centre of the muffin; if the skewer comes out clean, the muffins are ready.

Cool slightly in the tray and then turn muffins out on to a wire rack in their baking paper cases. Makes 12.

tip *Cool completely before storing in an airtight container. Muffins can also be individually wrapped in cling wrap and frozen.*

GOOD SOURCE OF: *low GI carbohydrate, vitamins C and B-group, calcium, folate, protein, potassium, magnesium, fibre*

GOOD FOR MOTHER: *constipation, calming and cleansing digestive system, fatigue, diabetes, healthy skin*

GOOD FOR BABY: *development of strong, healthy bones and nervous system, muscle contractions, formation of body fat, fuelling foetal growth*

214

Carrot and Hazelnut Muffins

These delicious muffins contain no added fat or sugar and are a nourishing way to satisfy sweet cravings. They also have a low GI rating to provide sustained energy. Take one to work for a nourishing snack.

1¼ cups self-raising wholemeal flour

2½ tsp mixed spice (or cinnamon and nutmeg)

½ cup skim milk powder

½ tsp baking powder

⅓ cup wheatgerm

⅓ cup hazelnuts, roughly chopped

½ cup (125 ml/4 fl oz) milk

1 cup (250 ml/8 fl oz) apple or pear juice

1 egg, lightly beaten

⅔ cup sultanas

2 cups finely grated carrot

Preheat oven to 180°C/350°F. Prepare a 12 cup muffin tray. Line bases with baking paper.

Sift flour, spices, skim milk powder and baking powder into a large mixing bowl. Tip the husk flakes remaining in the sifter into the bowl. Add wheatgerm and nuts and gently fold through.

In a separate bowl, combine milk, apple juice and the beaten egg.

Make a well in the centre of the dry ingredients and add the milk mixture. Gently fold through with a large metal spoon until *just* combined. Add the sultanas and grated carrot and again fold through a few times. Vigorous or over-mixing can result in a dense and heavy texture.

Spoon mixture into prepared muffin tins and bake for 15 minutes, or until cooked. Cool muffins slightly in the tray before transferring on to a wire rack in their baking paper cases.

Cool completely before storing in an airtight container in the cupboard for up to 3 days. Muffins are also suitable for freezing. Wrap muffins individually in freezer bags or cling wrap on the day of baking to capture the freshness. Remove as needed or take a frozen muffin to work in the morning and you will have a fresh muffin ready to eat by mid-morning. Makes 12.

215

GOOD SOURCE OF: *B-group vitamins including folate, calcium, zinc, beta-carotene, essential fatty acids, fibre*

GOOD FOR MOTHER: *constipation, heartburn, circulation, immunity, healthy skin, hair, nails, skin elasticity, hypertension, diabetes*

GOOD FOR BABY: *rapid foetal and cell growth, development of brain, eyes, immune and nervous systems, strong bone structure*

fRuit anD Nut BaRs

A great 'takeaway' snack, these bars can be baked and stored in an airtight container for up to 5–7 days, or frozen for later use. The skim milk powder makes this a high protein/calcium-rich snack, low in fat and rich in B-group vitamins that may prevent the onset of nausea.

1 cup figs, roughly chopped (or half figs/ half apricot for lower GI count)

1 cup pitted prunes, roughly chopped

1 cup (250 ml/8 fl oz) water

1 tbs cinnamon/mixed spice

½ tsp bicarbonate of soda

½ cup stoneground, wholemeal plain flour

2 tbs skim milk powder

½ cup rolled oats

½ cup almonds, roughly chopped

½ cup each sunflower seeds, sesame seeds and pepitas

1 egg, lightly beaten

Preheat oven to 160°C/325°F. Line a 27 x 17 cm shallow baking tin with baking paper.

Place chopped dried fruit, water and spices in a small saucepan. Bring to boil, then reduce heat to a simmer. Cover and cook for 2–3 minutes. Add bicarbonate of soda and stir to combine. Remove from heat and set aside, leaving lid on.

Sift flour and skim milk powder into a large mixing bowl. Add oats, nuts, seeds and warm dried fruit mixture. Combine all ingredients.

Lightly beat egg in a separate bowl. Add to mixture and mix well. Pour mixture into the prepared baking tin. Spread evenly across the base of the tin by pressing down with the back of a spoon or the heel of your hand.

Bake for 10–15 minutes, or until golden brown. Remove from oven and cool in baking tin. Cut into 3 x 6 cm squares. Makes 20 squares.

tip *Most dried fruit contains preservative 220 (sulphur). This preserves the fruit and often gives it its colour (preservative-free dried apricots are almost black in colour, rather than bright orange!) Organic dried fruit is sold in all good health food stores or online at www.goodness.com.au*

GOOD SOURCE OF: protein, calcium, magnesium, potassium, essential fatty acids, fibre, vitamins K and B-group, antioxidants, moderate amounts of iron and zinc

GOOD FOR MOTHER: fatigue, constipation, skin elasticity, hypertension, leg cramps, nausea, nourishing uterus, hormone production, increased blood supply, fertility

GOOD FOR BABY: strong bones, healthy skin, hair and eyes, steady heartbeat, development of brain and nervous system, general foetal growth

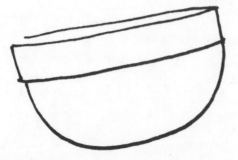

Choc, Fruit and Nut Balls

Satisfy a chocolate craving with these wholesome fruit balls. Good quality cocoa is rich in iron and doesn't contain the fat and sugar of processed chocolate. Dried fruit adds natural sweetness, nuts add nourishment and the skim milk powder boosts protein and calcium intake. The challenge of this recipe is not to eat the mixture during preparation! It is also the perfect opportunity to have some fun with young children in the kitchen. Ask them to help roll up the balls. But be warned, there will be sticky fingers!

⅓ cup cocoa

½ cup skim milk powder

⅓ cup (80 ml/2¾ fl oz) boiling water

⅔ cup (100 g) natural almonds, roughly chopped

⅓ cup pepitas

1 tbs sesame seeds

½ cup (100 g) dried apricots, roughly chopped

½ cup (50 g) sultanas

½ cup (50 g) prunes, pitted and roughly chopped

Line an airtight container with baking paper or a paper towel.

Mix cocoa, skim milk powder and boiling water in a small cup and stir until smooth.

Dry roast almonds in a frying pan. Place roasted almonds in a food processor and blend until finely chopped. Pour half of the almonds into a bowl and set aside. Leave the other half in the food processor.

Add pepitas, sesame seeds and dried fruit to the food processor and process until well combined. Add cocoa mixture and blend once more.

Spread the remaining almonds on a plate or board. With damp hands, roll teaspoons of the mixture into balls. Roll balls in the almonds to coat.

Place in prepared container and chill to store. Makes 24.

tip *Store in the fridge for up to one week . . . if they last that long! Also suitable for freezing.*

GOOD SOURCE OF: *protein, calcium, magnesium, potassium, iron, essential fatty acids, zinc, B-group vitamins, fibre*

GOOD FOR MOTHER: *sweet cravings, fatigue, healthy skin, constipation, anaemia, kidney function, production of colostrum and red blood cells, immunity, healthy heart*

GOOD FOR BABY: *development of muscles, bones, brain and central nervous system, eyesight*

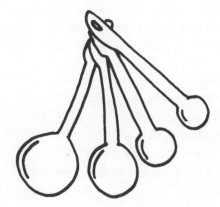

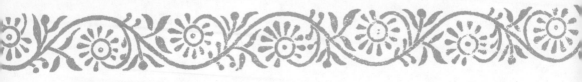

❀ ways with bread

Bread is such a versatile snack, perfect for breakfast, between meals or for a late night supper. Start with a wholesome base and a healthy spread and you will be off to a great start. Pile toppings high on wholegrain toast, or pack nourishing fillings into sandwiches. For simpler fare, who can resist a cheese and tomato melt, or good old Vegemite or Marmite on toast, often a great option when nauseous.

Choose from multi and mixed grain, soy and linseed, cape seed, spelt, sourdough and rye varieties as well as barley, rice and buckwheat breads for gluten-free alternatives. Wholemeal bread is a healthy option, but has a higher GI rating. Breads with visible grains provide a more sustained energy source.

sandwich fillings

The sandwich would have to be the most popular portable food of western civilisation. This portability makes is ideal for the pregnancy diet. There will be times when you will be out and about and suddenly overcome by hunger. With nothing but undesirable takeaway choices available, having a Vegemite or cheese sandwich in your handbag will be a godsend. Don't leave home without one!

Sandwiches are also an easy way to double your nutrient intake. Think of how many different ingredients you can pack into just one sandwich. Up to ten ingredients go into my favourite chicken and salad roll. And you can substitute butter and margarine with nutritionally rich spreads such as avocado, hummus, pesto and low-fat cottage and cream cheeses.

Filling options are endless and can be created to suit individual tastes. Choose from open or closed sandwiches, rolls, baguettes, wraps and pita bread pockets. Start with a high protein source and then load it up with fresh, raw vegetables. The following suggestions are easy to make at home, pre-pack for work or order from a sandwich bar.

- beef: Pesto, tomato, baby rocket leaves

    Grilled eggplant, hummus, baby spinach leaves

    Roast beef, mustard, tomato and cheese

    steak sandwich

- canned salmon: Avocado, rocket, spring onions, coriander or parsley. (*Mash* avocado and combine with salmon. Mix with diced spring onions, rocket and herbs. Finish with a squeeze of lime juice and black pepper)

Cucumber, baby spinach leaves and low-fat cream cheese

Boiled egg, tomato, red onion and mixed leaves

- canned tuna: Hummus and tabouleh wrapped in lavish or mountain bread

Mashed sweet potato and spring onions with avocado spread or cream cheese

Pesto, baby rocket leaves, cherry or semi-roasted tomatoes

Avocado, parsley and pepper

Rocket, avocado and hard cheese

Tasty Tuna Patties (see recipe) with yoghurt and mixed salad leaves

- chicken: Avocado, tomato, baby spinach leaves

Beetroot, cottage cheese and mixed leaves

Wrap with the works—hummus, avocado, carrot, beetroot, capsicum, cucumber, tomato, rocket, red onion—on mountain or lavish bread

- cheese: Edam, cheddar or tasty cheese on soy & linseed bread

Cottage cheese and salad

Cheese, lettuce and mustard. (Spread with your favourite mustard, top with a slice of hard cheese and finish with dark salad leaves, baby rocket or a micro herb and salad mix)

- vegetarian: Hummus and tabouli

Avocado, spinach, semi-roasted tomato and toasted nut mix

Pesto and roast vegetable. (Fill wholemeal pita bread with any of the following roast veges—tofu, eggplant, zucchini, red capsicum, tomato, mushroom—with hard cheese and fresh basil leaves)

- egg: Mash boiled egg with cottage cheese, top with watercress or dark salad leaves

Curried egg and baby spinach leaves

Toast toppings

These toppings have been devised to provide maximum goodness. They are easy to create at home, at work or ordered from a café or sandwich bar. If you want to create your own toppings, refer to the pregnancy superfoods as a guide to nourishing ingredients. Here are some of my suggestions:

- roast tomato, rocket and hummus on rye—spread rye toast generously with hummus, top with semi-roasted roma tomatoes and baby rocket leaves and serve with a smoothie for a balanced meal
- avocado, tomato and basil on spelt—spread avocado, and top with tomato and season with black pepper and fresh basil
- mushrooms on soy and linseed—sauté button mushrooms in a little olive oil and garlic then season with black pepper and fresh parsley. Spread toast with avocado or hummus and top with mushrooms
- cheese and Vegemite melt on wholegrain—spread toast with Vegemite and top with a slice of tasty cheese and melt under the grill. Rich in calcium and the B-group vitamins
- tuna and cheese toastie—combine 110 g (4 oz) canned tuna with grated cheese and baby spinach leaves or finely diced green capsicum. Make a sandwich with the filling and cook in a sandwich maker until golden brown. Multi-grain bread boosts the omega 3 properties of this snack, recommended for the third trimester
- hummus and roasted veg on sourdough—lightly toast sourdough and spread with hummus and pile high with roasted vegetables, including capsicum, zucchini, mushrooms, tomatoes and fresh herbs. Perfect use for leftovers
- boiled eggs, mashed with pepper and a tablespoon of finely chopped parsley or chives
- avocado with a squeeze of lemon juice, salt and pepper
- vegemite
- natural peanut butter (available from health food stores)
- cheese and tomato open grill
- fruit spread (*see recipe*).

Egg Pesto

Basil and eggs taste wonderful together and are equally nutritious, so I have combined two classic versions of each: the boiled egg and pesto. Good quality pesto is easy to find these days but you can also whip up a chunky pesto spread in a flash with the use of a mortar and pestle.

> 1 boiled egg
>
> pesto (homemade or good quality bought)
>
> 2 slices wholegrain toast

Boil egg. Make pesto (see below).

Generously spread toast with pesto. Slice or mash the eggs and arrange on top. Delicious! Serves 1.

Chunky Pesto Spread

> ½ firmly packed cup fresh basil leaves
>
> 1 small clove garlic, roughly chopped
>
> ½ cup almonds or brazil nuts
>
> 1 tbs parmesan cheese, finely grated
>
> 2 tsp extra virgin olive oil
>
> cracked black pepper

I use a mortar and pestle as I love the rustic result. A food processor can also be used—just be sure not to over-process. This pesto should have a chunky texture.

Pound or process basil, then add garlic to form a paste. Add the nuts and parmesan cheese and briefly pound/process for a chunky texture.

Drizzle 1 teaspoon of olive oil over the mixture and stir with a spoon if using a mortar and pestle, or on low speed if in a processor. The oil will bring the ingredients together to form our pesto spread. Add a little more oil if needed and season with cracked black pepper to taste.

Sardines on Toast

Sardines are nourishing little nippers for both you and your baby, They are an excellent source of omega 3, with a small tin providing more than the daily recommended intake. Sardines are also a great source of iodine and calcium, so think brain and bone food. Parsley and lemon balance their strong flavour and when topped on some wholesome bread this is a delicious snack. Refer to my *Red Capsicums Stuffed with Sardines* receipe for another yummy way to enjoy the goodness of sardines.

> 1 small tin sardines in springwater
>
> 1–2 tbs fresh parsley, chopped
>
> juice of ½ lemon
>
> cracked black pepper
>
> 2 slices toast (spelt bread is wonderful with this recipe)
>
> avocado to serve

Combine sardines, parsley and lemon juice in a bowl. Season with black pepper. Cook toast, spread generously with avocado and spoon sardine mixture on top. Serves 1.

GOOD SOURCE OF: *omega 3, iodine, calcium, protein, iron, vitamins C, E and B-group, antioxidants, fibre*

GOOD FOR MOTHER: *skin elasticity, healthy uterus, skin and hair, constipation, lactation, reducing risk of osteoporosis, aiding kidney function*

GOOD FOR BABY: *rapid foetal growth, brain and nerve development, strong bones, teeth and nails, muscle contractions, including heartbeat*

Pears on Toast

We all have occasional sweet cravings. This is a cleansing way to start the day for breakfast, or just as good as an afternoon snack. Pears are wonderful for digestion and have a very low GI rating suitable for diabetics. Stewed pears only take minutes to prepare and can be used in a number of dishes or as a quick snack.

    2 stewed/canned pear halves, sliced

    2 thick slices sourdough toast

    low-fat cottage or cream cheese

    2 strawberries, sliced

    1 fresh mint leaf, shredded (optional)

Prepare the pears. Lightly toast the bread. Spread toast with the cheese, layer the pears then the strawberries and finish with a few shredded pieces of fresh mint.

225

tip *To stew pears, place thinly sliced pears in a saucepan with ½ cup (125 ml/ 4 fl oz) of water. Cover and simmer for 3 to 4 minutes, until just tender. Store with juices in an airtight container in the refrigerator.*

Spiced Banana Jaffle

This is like a mini banana pie and the freshly grated nutmeg is absolutely delicious.

    1 banana, mashed

    ¼ cup low-fat cottage cheese

    pinch of nutmeg

    2 slices wholegrain bread

Combine the mashed banana and cottage cheese and sprinkle with nutmeg. Make into a sandwich and then toast in a sandwich maker for a sweet, creamy delight.

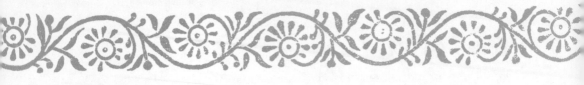

❁ Sides

These side dishes are to accompany your fish, chicken, meat or vegetarian protein sources, but they can also serve as healthy snacks. Most are rich in vitamin C, which will increase iron absorption, and folate, which works best when combined with vitamin B12, found in protein-rich foods. These sides can be eaten throughout the entire pregnancy, but I have nominated a trimester where particular dishes may be most beneficial.

Salsas

Salsas are a delicious way to flavour foods with natural, healthy ingredients and make the most of fresh herbs. Mint, coriander, parsley and basil all work well in salsas. Salsas are fabulous with all meats and fish, either served as a side or as a filling for a wrap or tortilla. Of course there are nutritional benefits to this combo, too. Salsas are always rich in vitamin C, so eating them with first class protein such as meat increases iron absorption. Salsas look so impressive and yet take less than five minutes to make. They do benefit if left to stand for ten minutes for flavours to develop. Make the salsa first it will be ready by the time you prepare the accompanying dish.

Summer Salsa

Perfect on fish or chicken.

> 2 nectarines or peaches
>
> ½ red capsicum, finely diced
>
> ½ avocado, finely diced
>
> 2 shallots, finely diced
>
> 2 tbs fresh mint leaves, finely shredded
>
> juice of 1 lime

Combine all ingredients in a bowl. Set aside for 10 minutes.

Mango Salsa

This is probably the most versatile salsa as it complements fish and all white and red meats.

1 mango, diced

½ red capsicum, diced

1 cucumber, diced

½ red onion, diced

½ cup fresh coriander, chopped

juice of 1 lime

cracked black pepper

Combine all the ingredients in a bowl and season with black pepper. Rest for 10 minutes before serving.

Tomato Salsa

Great with steak, on a steak sandwich or tossed through warm pasta with sliced chicken breast.

2 tomatoes, finely diced

½ red onion

2 tbs basil

1 tsp olive oil

1 small clove garlic, optional

cracked black pepper

small pinch iodised salt

Combine all ingredients in a bowl. Set aside for 10 minutes.

Corn Salsa

The perfect complement to Moroccan spiced foods.

1 corn cob, cooked, kernels removed

100g (3½ oz) green beans, very finely sliced

1 red capsicum, finely diced

½ red onion, finely diced

½ bunch coriander, chopped

1 avocado, diced

juice of 1 lime

cracked black pepper

227

Combine the ingredients in a bowl. Set aside for 10 minutes prior to serving.

Papaya Salsa

Fantastic on grilled chicken breast or with barbeque prawns and scallops.

½ papaya, deseeded and finely diced

½ tsp red chilli, finely diced

1 shallot, finely chopped

1 tbs fresh mint

juice of ½ lime

Combine all ingredients in a bowl. Set aside for 10 minutes.

Spring vegetables

Boost your folate levels and revive your taste buds. This side works with any meat, chicken or fish dish, or on its own as a nourishing snack. Your baby will love you for it. Select no less than five of the vegetables, with at least one being asparagus, broccoli or Brussels sprouts.

asparagus

broccoli

cauliflower

Brussels sprouts

peas

green beans

sugar snap or snow peas

fresh corn cob, cut into small lengths

English spinach leaves

dressing:

2 tbs flaxseed oil

1 tbs apple cider vinegar

1 clove garlic, crushed

cracked black pepper

Combine all dressing ingredients and vigorously whisk or shake together.

Wash and trim vegetables. Steam in a steamer saucepan the more robust vegetables first, adding the more fragile varieties towards the end: corn (6–8 minutes), Brussels sprouts and cauliflower (5 minutes), broccoli, beans and peas (3 minutes), asparagus and spinach (2 minutes) and snow peas, sugar snap peas and spinach no longer than one minute.

Remove from the steamer and pour the dressing into the warm saucepan. Return the vegetables to the pan and gently shake to coat with the dressing. Tip into a serving bowl along with any excess dressing in the saucepan.

GOOD SOURCE OF: *folate, vitamins A, C and K, potassium, magnesium, fibre*

GOOD FOR MOTHER: *preconception, immune system, constipation, healthy skin, good health*

GOOD FOR BABY: *development of brain, spine, genetic material and central nervous system, reducing risk of birth defects, supporting rapid cell and organ growth, strong bone structure*

wok-tossed Vegetables

The trick to perfect wok-tossed vegetables is to work very quickly in a hot wok. This delivers firm but tender veges and reduces cooking time and loss of nutrients. This dish also serves as a snack with a bowl of brown rice.

1 bunch bok choy, leaves separated

1 bunch broccolini or 1 medium head of broccoli

1 small red capsicum

½ bunch garlic sprouts

3 shallots, sliced diagonally

2 garlic cloves, crushed

2 cm ginger, peeled and sliced into thin strips

1 tsp sesame seeds

1 tbs water

1 tbs oyster sauce

1 tbs grape seed oil

229

Wash and prepare all vegetables, spices and seeds. Combine the water and oyster sauce in a small jug and mix to combine.

Heat oil in a hot wok. Add ginger and garlic and stir-fry for 30 seconds. Add red capsicum, garlic sprouts, broccolini and bok choy. Stir-fry for one minute before pouring over the oyster sauce and water. Continue cooking for 2–3 minutes, or until vegetables are firm but tender. Finally, stir through shallots. Transfer into a serving bowl and sprinkle with sesame seeds.

GOOD SOURCE OF: *vitamins A, C and K, folate, calcium, antioxidants, potassium, fibre*

GOOD FOR MOTHER: *preconception, fatigue, digestion, circulation, immunity, healthy placenta and uterus, iron absorption, normal blood clotting, converting food to fuel*

GOOD FOR BABY: *reducing risk of birth defects, proper development of neural tube and central nervous system, cell growth, eyesight, strong bones and teeth*

steameD GReens with NouRishing Nut Mix

This dish is fantastic during the first trimester for the initial development of the neural tube. However, I recommend you continue eating it throughout your pregnancy to complete development. Folate is best absorbed when eaten with foods rich in vitamin B12, so serve this with meat, chicken, fish or eggs.

100 g (3½ oz) brussels sprouts, trimmed and halved

1 small head of broccoli, cut into bite-size florets

100 g (3½ oz) green beans, trimmed and halved

1 bunch asparagus

small handful sugar snap peas

½ cup nourishing nut and seed mix (see page ?)

flaxseed oil

Prepare a medium-large steamer and bring water to the boil. Add brussels sprouts and steam for 3 minutes. Add broccoli, beans and asparagus and continue steaming for 2 minutes. Add sugar snap peas and blanch for a final 30–60 seconds. All vegetables, with the exception of the brussels sprouts, should be just firm but tender, with a slight crunch.

Immediately transfer vegetables into a serving bowl. Add nut and seed mixture and drizzle with 1 teaspoon of flaxseed oil. Season with cracked black pepper if desired.

GOOD SOURCE OF: *folate, vitamins A, C, K and B-group, calcium, potassium, essential fatty acids, fibre, protein, zinc*

GOOD FOR MOTHER: *preconception, fertility, immunity, strong blood capillaries, healthy placenta, skin elasticity, red blood cell production when eaten with vitamin B12*

GOOD FOR BABY: *normal development of neural tube, brain and eyes, strong bones, teeth and nails, muscle coordination, organ and cell growth*

Ginger and Lemon Roasted Carrots

Carrots are one of the only vegetables that are more nutritious when cooked. This is a great dish to have if you feel the onset of a cold or flu, with ginger and lemons age-old remedies.

4 carrots

2 tsp olive oil

1 tbs lemon

1 tsp finely grated ginger

cracked black pepper

Preheat oven to 180°C/350°F. Line a baking tray with baking paper.

Cut carrots into chunky sticks. Whisk together oil, lemon juice, ginger and cracked black pepper in an airtight container. Add carrots, place lid on the container and shake to coat evenly.

Pour carrots and marinade on to the baking tray and bake for 30 minutes.

231

tip *If short on time, steam the carrots for 5 minutes, or until just tender. Toss the warm carrots in the marinade and then bake for 15 minutes until golden brown.*

GOOD SOURCE OF: *beta-carotene, antioxidants*

GOOD FOR MOTHER: *nausea, heartburn, constipation, flatulence, circulation, helping to fight infection, healing wounds, increasing red blood cell count*

GOOD FOR BABY: *development of cells, eyes, healthy hair, skin and nails*

Tomato and Basil Salad

Tomatoes are extremely rich in antioxidants and absorption is enhanced when combined with olive oil. Their vitamin C content maxmises iron absorption and so is the perfect partner to iron-rich dishes. The cleansing flavours of this salad are the perfect barbeque accompaniment, especially with our *Mediterranean Steaks*.

½ punnet each of red and yellow cherry or grape tomatoes, halved

½ red onion, finely diced

6 large basil leaves, shredded

1 tsp extra virgin olive oil

cracked black pepper

Toss all ingredients into a bowl. Rest the salad at room temperature for 5 minutes before serving.

232

GOOD SOURCE OF: *beta-carotene, vitamins C and E, omega 3 and 6, antioxidants*

GOOD FOR MOTHER: *healthy heart, teeth and gums, supple skin, strengthening immune system, hypertension, fluid retention, nourishing uterus and placenta, iron absorption, postnatal recovery, lactation*

GOOD FOR BABY: *protecting against cell damage, eyesight, muscle contractions, strong teeth and bones*

Bean, Spinach and Avocado Salad with Poppy Seed Dressing

This salad promotes excellent health and is great for baby's overall growth. Tomato, spinach and avocado should always be eaten together as the combination releases the antioxidants contained in each. Team this salad with beef, lamb, chicken, fish or tofu and maximise iron absorption.

100 g (3½ oz) green beans

2 tomatoes, quartered

½ avocado, sliced

1 lebanese cucumber, sliced diagonally

1 cup baby spinach leaves

poppy seed vinaigrette:

1 tbs extra virgin olive oil

2 tsp cider vinegar

1 tsp lemon juice

1 tsp black poppy seeds

cracked black pepper

very small pinch sea salt

233

Trim the beans and lightly steam for 1–2 minutes. Allow to cool while you prepare the salad. Combine the olive oil, vinegar, lemon juice, poppy seeds and seasonings in a small cup and whisk together. Prepare all remaining ingredients and toss into a salad bowl. Add beans and dressing.

GOOD SOURCE OF: *omega 3, vitamins C, E, K and B-group especially folate and B6, beta-carotene, fibre, potassium, magnesium, antioxidants*

GOOD FOR MOTHER: *fluid retention, leg cramps, digestion, dental problems, healthy skin, hair and bones, skin elasticity, healthy uterus, healing and tissue repair, fatigue, hypertension*

GOOD FOR BABY: *growth of healthy cells, eyesight, brain development, strong bone and cell structure*

Mushroom, Red Capsicum and Green Bean Salad

This salad is bursting with vitamin C and B-group vitamins and is particularly beneficial when served with a high-protein source. Iron absorption and the function of vitamin B12 are enhanced for healthy blood and less chance of developing anaemia. Mushrooms are a useful source of protein and vitamin B12 on their own, so this is a wise choice for vegetarians.

1 tbs flaxseed or extra virgin olive oil

1 tbs balsamic vinegar

cracked black pepper

100 g (3½ oz) button mushrooms

100 g (3½ oz) green beans, cut into 2 cm lengths

½ red capsicum, diced

2 shallots, finely diced

1 tbs chopped parsley

234

Combine oil, vinegar and black pepper in a medium bowl. Whisk to combine.

Thoroughly remove any excess dirt from the mushrooms. Cut into quarters and toss through the dressing in the bowl. Allow to marinate while you prepare salad ingredients.

Lightly steam the beans and add to the mushrooms with all remaining ingredients.

Toss together and serve.

GOOD SOURCE OF: *vitamins C, E, B2, B5 and B12, folate, beta-carotene, omega 3, phosphorus, potassium*

GOOD FOR MOTHER: *vegetarians, fatigue, circulation, fluid retention, skin elasticity, lactation, healthy blood, nourishing placenta, supporting immune system of both mother and baby*

GOOD FOR BABY: *development of brain and genetic material, eyesight, converting food to fuel*

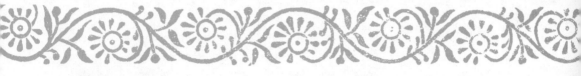

❄ Drinks

Drinks are perfect for pregnancy and lactation. They are a quick and easy way to consume essential nutrients as well as hydrating the body. A few ingredients tossed into a blender create a healthy fix in under five minutes.

Blender drinks come in the form of milkshakes, smoothies and frappes and are easily digested by the body. There are a variety of blender drink recipes to choose from in this book but the choices of other combinations are endless. Please note all drink recipes serve 1. Below is a list of good fruits for pregnancy that are great additions or substitutes for any blender drink. Because you are using raw ingredients for these, make sure you wash them well before using.

RICH IN FOLATE	RICH IN VITAMIN C	LOW GI RATING
papaya	all berries	pears
oranges	guava	berries
kiwi fruit	kiwi fruit	apricots
strawberries	mango	plums
bananas	papaya	peaches and nectarines
rockmelon	pineapple	bananas (when not overripe)

Milkshakes and smoothies are dairy rich and a fabulous source of protein and calcium. Frappes are dairy-free and are rich in folate and vitamin C. Frappes are a blend of fruit and ice, or fruit and frozen fruit, and they are refreshing and very hydrating. I have provided a 'base' recipe that can be enjoyed as is, or with different seasonal fruits for added flavour and nutrients. Frappes do need to be served immediately to prevent ingredients from separating.

Fresh juices are best consumed in the morning, on an empty stomach, for maximum nutritional absorption. I always drink my juice immediately after juicing as nutrients are lost as soon as you start washing, peeling or cutting fruit and vegetables. Freshly squeezed juices should be consumed within six hours and stored in the refrigerator until use. It is also advised to wait one hour after drinking your juice before consuming tea or coffee. Caffeinated products can inhibit the absorption of all that goodness. The general rule when creating your own juice combinations is five parts vegetables to one part fruit. Fruit should really only be included to sweeten the juice. If you can go without fruit, great, but never hold back with the vegetables. Despite the amazing benefits of juices, they should not be used as a complete substitute for whole, fresh raw fruit and vegetables as a good part of dietary fibre is lost during juicing.

Tea Infusions are an effective way to make use of the therapeutic and healing properties of herbs and spices. They cleanse, calm and revive the body, or can help to relieve digestive problems, cold and flu symptoms and nausea. Drinking hot tea or coffee with breakfast may interfere with digestion. Hot liquid and the tannin found in tea are not favourable to bacteria, especially the kind found in yoghurt. Try to delay drinking hot drinks an hour before or after eating yoghurt.

236

Vitamin C Crush

For your second trimester but drink throughout your pregnancy. I have used pineapple and kiwi fruit in this frappe for their incredibly high vitamin C content, keeping you and your baby very healthy. This juice is also fabulous for digestion, with pears, pineapple and mint all aiding the process.

½ cup (125 ml/4 fl oz) unsweetened pineapple juice

1 kiwi fruit, peeled and roughly chopped

½ pear, roughly chopped

5 ice cubes

fresh mint leaves (optional)

Blend all ingredients until thick and creamy. Serve immediately.

Berry Blast

Great for preconception and first trimester. Enjoy my Berry Blast for breakfast, between meals or even as a dessert. It is rich in antioxidants to boost the immune system and prime your body for the nine months ahead. A great meal option when nauseous and solids are hard to tolerate.

1 banana

½ cup berries

3–4 ice cubes

⅓ cup (80 ml/2¾ fl oz) skim milk/soy milk

1 tbs skim milk powder

½ cup plain yoghurt/soy yoghurt

1 tbs wheatgerm

Place fruit and ice into blender and process for 30 seconds.

Add remaining ingredients and blend until smooth.

237

GOOD SOURCE OF: *calcium, protein, antioxidants, potassium, vitamin C, zinc, folate, essential fatty acids*

GOOD FOR MOTHER: *digestion, loss of appetite, fertility, healthy kidneys and uterus, leg cramps, boostings immune system, production of collagen for skin elasticity, hypertension, growing placenta*

GOOD FOR BABY: *overall foetal development including major organs and circulatory systems, resuming and regulating heartbeat, production of genetic material and healthy body cells, strong teeth, skin, nails, development of eyes, leg cramps*

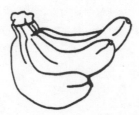

Banana and Ginger Milkshake

Give this a go during the first and second trimesters. This sounds like a strange combination for a milkshake but it is surprisingly yummy. It may assist in relieving morning sickness and is particularly good for those who cannot tolerate solids and/or protein. Milkshakes are easy to digest and meet a substantial quota of your nutritional daily requirements, which are usually compromised when nauseous. The fresh ginger and nutmeg are known to relieve nausea and the yoghurt will aid digestion. The combination of magnesium-rich bananas and calcium-rich milk should assist with leg cramps.

1 ripe banana

1 cup (250 ml/8 fl oz) low-fat milk/soy milk

½ cup low-fat plain yoghurt/soy yoghurt

1 tsp finely grated fresh ginger root

½ tsp finely grated fresh nutmeg

4 ice cubes

Place all ingredients into a blender and process until thick and creamy.

tip *Fresh nutmeg is worth a try and is known to ease nausea. The flavour is quite different and just delicious. Try it freshly grated over cooked spinach, roast pumpkin or with desserts made with banana or ginger and honey.*

GOOD SOURCE OF: *protein, calcium, potassium, magnesium, vitamins A, D, B12 and folate*

GOOD FOR MOTHER: *nausea, circulation, digestion, leg cramps, complete and proper calcium function*

GOOD FOR BABY: *strong bones, teeth and skeletal structure, healthy skin, hair and eyes, brain/nerve/muscle coordination, production of genetic material and red blood cells*

TROPiCaL DeLight

For your third trimester and during lactation. This smoothie delivers more than twice the recommended daily requirement of vitamin C, an important nutrient throughout pregnancy and lactation. It is a great energy source to fight fatigue and provides the essential nutrients for the final phases of foetal growth and development.

1 cup (250 ml/8 fl oz) low-fat milk/low-fat soy milk

½ medium papaya, flesh only

1 banana

juice of ½ fresh lime

Place all ingredients into a blender and process until smooth. Pour into a glass with a few ice cubes.

GOOD SOURCE OF: *vitamins A and C, fibre, potassium, calcium, folate*

GOOD FOR MOTHER: *dental hygiene, healthy skin/stretch marks, fatigue, leg cramps, constipation and diarrhoea, hypertension, production of collagen, healthy placenta and uterus*

GOOD FOR BABY: *healthy skin, hair and eyes for both mother and baby, development of immune and nervous systems*

239

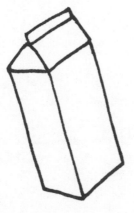

Mango smoothie

Good throughout pregnancy and during lactation, particularly your second trimester. It is an added bonus that delicious tropical fruits such as the mango are crammed with nutrition. Mangoes, yoghurt and milk are a great combination and, with the wheatgerm, this smoothie pretty much provides most of your daily pregnancy nutritional needs. Enjoy with breakfast, or as a nourishing snack at any time of the day. The high content of vitamin C makes this smoothie fabulous during lactation.

> 1 cup mango
>
> handful ice cubes
>
> ½ cup (125 ml/4 fl oz) low-fat milk or soy milk
>
> ½ cup low-fat plain or soy yoghurt
>
> 1 tbs wheatgerm

Place mango flesh and ice cubes in a blender and process for a couple of seconds. Add all remaining ingredients and blend until smooth and creamy.

tip *One mango provides more than the daily recommended dose of vitamin C, more than half the recommended dose of vitamins A and E, as well as being a useful source of iron, potassium and fibre. Mangoes also contain enzymes that help to break down protein for the body to use more effectively. Indulge and enjoy.*

GOOD SOURCE OF: *vitamins C, A, E and B12, folate, fibre, potassium, calcium, protein, antioxidants*

GOOD FOR MOTHER: *immune system, skin elasticity, hypertension, fatigue, sustained energy source, circulation/varicose veins, hormone production, lactation, helping postnatal recovery*

GOOD FOR BABY: *healthy foetal growth and development, especially brain, teeth, skin and bones, eyesight, cell reproduction, brain/muscle coordination*

full-o-folate frappe

Particularly for the first trimester but great throughout your pregnancy. As the title suggests, this is full of folate, together with vitamins C and B6, potassium and fibre. It may assist with fatigue, leg cramps, constipation, hypertension and is excellent for the digestive tract. Use this as your basic frappe recipe.

> ½ cup (125 ml/4 fl oz) freshly squeezed orange juice
>
> 1 large banana
>
> 1 cup ice cubes

Blend all ingredients until thick and creamy. Serve immediately.

tip   *Add any one of the following to the basic frappe recipe: ½ mango, diced (rich in vitamins A, C, E and fibre); 1 cup fresh strawberries (rich source of folate and vitamin C); ½ cup frozen blueberries (excellent source of vitamin C and powerful antioxidant); ½ cup diced papaya (folate-rich).*

241

feeling nauseous

Try this during first trimester. Many expecting mums claim sour-tasting foods can often help with nausea. The tangy flavours of green apple and lime may assist.

1 green apple	OR	1 green apple
½ fresh lime, skin removed		½ cup fresh fennel
2 cm knob fresh ginger		2 cm knob fresh ginger
handful fresh mint leaves		

Feed all ingredients through juicer. Stir to combine before drinking.

GOOD SOURCE OF: *vitamin C, pectin*

GOOD FOR MOTHER: *nausea, circulation, digestion, stimulating appetite, cleansing, helping eliminate heavy metals from the body*

Berry Delights

Berries are extremely rich in antioxidants and vitamin C, which strengthen the immune system, guard against cell damage, nourish the placenta and keep you in excellent health. A wide range of frozen berries are now available in supermarkets. They are frozen fresh and have absolutely no added sugar or preservatives, making them ideal for our Berry Delights.

Berry one:

½ cup frozen blueberries

1 banana

½ cup (125 ml/4 fl oz) freshly squeezed orange juice

6 ice cubes

Berry two:

1 cup mixed berries

1 cup (250 ml/8 fl oz) freshly squeezed orange juice

4 ice cubes

Berry three:

½ cup frozen raspberries

1 pear, cored and diced

½ cup (125 ml/4 fl oz) freshly squeezed orange juice

3 ice cubes

Berry four:

1 cup frozen forest fruit berries or summer berries

1 cup (250 ml/8 fl oz) pear or apple juice (freshly juiced, or if purchased no sugar)

Place ingredients in a blender and process until smooth.

242

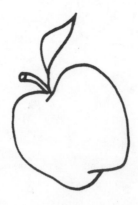

Energy and Immune Boost Juice

Great for first and third trimesters. This is an antioxidant-rich juice, fantastic for the immune system to help heal and fight off infection. It is also fantastic for the blood. Beetroot is known to increase the uptake of oxygen in the blood. This oxygen is circulated around the body, generating energy for you and nourishing the placenta.

> 2 carrots
>
> ½ medium apple
>
> ½ medium beetroot
>
> 1 stick celery
>
> 2 cm piece fresh ginger

Feed all ingredients through juicer. Stir to combine before drinking.

GOOD SOURCE OF: *beta-carotene, vitamin C, fibre, antioxidants*

GOOD FOR MOTHER: *immune system, fighting off infection, general good health, cleansing the liver, activating digestion, blood circulation, anaemia, fatigue, fluid retention, nausea, hypertension, healthy skin, eyes, hair and nails*

Digestive Tonic

For first and second trimesters. Pears are known for their healing and calming properties and are especially helpful for digestion and healthy bowel function.

> 2 pears
>
> 2 cm knob fresh ginger
>
> handful of fresh mint leaves

Feed all ingredients through juicer. Stir to combine before drinking.

GOOD SOURCE OF: *vitamins C and A, potassium, low GI rating*

GOOD FOR MOTHER: *nausea, constipation, fatigue, digestion, reflux and heartburn*

COLD AND FLU TONIC

Drink any time throughout pregnancy. This juice is famous at The Golden Door Health Retreat for its healing properties. During pregnancy, consider this your cold and flu tonic. Don't be deterred by the combination of ingredients. The honey and parsley act to neutralise the strong flavours that will ward off any nasty bugs or viruses. You don't have to be suffering from a cold or flu to reap the benefits of this juice. It is a great pick-me-up and promotes excellent health. As with all juices, this is most effective in the morning on an empty stomach.

2 oranges, juiced

1 lemon, juiced

2 cm piece fresh ginger, chopped

1 clove garlic, chopped

pinch of chilli (optional)

1 tsp manuka honey

handful of fresh parsley

Place all ingredients into a blender and blend together. Serve immediately.

Thanks to The Golden Door, Australia.

GOOD SOURCE OF: *vitamin C, beta-carotene, antioxidants*

GOOD FOR MOTHER: *strengthening immune system, resisting infection, relieving colds and flu symptoms, healthy heart, blood circulation, hypertension, good health*

Green Giant

A must for first trimester. A great morning energiser that contains all the goodness of raw spinach which is high in folate. The tangy flavours may appeal to those suffering from nausea.

1 cup English spinach leaves

1 green apple

juice of ½ lemon

6–8 mint leaves

Feed spinach and apple through juicer at medium speed. Reduce to low speed and add lemon and mint. Stir to combine ingredients before drinking.

GOOD SOURCE OF: *vitamins A, C, E and K, folate, potassium, magnesium*

GOOD FOR MOTHER: *strengthening immune system, muscle contractions, healthy skin and hair, constipation, hormone production, excellent health*

GOOD FOR BABY: *proper development of brain and neural tube, reducing risk of birth defects, supporting rapid cell growth, production of genetic material*

245

Body Cleanser

Drink throughout pregnancy. A cleansing juice that is beneficial to treating nausea.

2 carrots

1 orange

2 cm knob ginger

Feed all ingredients through juicer. Stir to combine before drinking.

GOOD SOURCE OF: *vitamin C, beta-carotene*

GOOD FOR MOTHER: *healthy skin, hair, circulatory systems and eyesight, helping to eliminate toxic wastes, boosting immune system, promoting cell growth*

Cleansing Tea

Activates the digestive system to flush out toxins, especially if consumed on an empty stomach in the morning. It is also good for nausea, blood circulation and for keeping colds and flu at bay.

3–4 slices fresh ginger

½ lemon, thinly sliced

6 mint leaves

Place all ingredients in a large mug or small teapot. Fill with boiling water and infuse for 3–5 minutes.

Uplifting Tea

A zingy tea that will both energise and refresh. Try it as a substitute for caffeine.

3–4 slices fresh ginger

⅓ stalk fresh lemongrass

Cut lemongrass into 3 cm pieces and bend slightly to bruise and release flavours. Place all ingredients in a large mug or small teapot. Add boiling water and infuse for 3–5 minutes.

Digesting Tea

Fennel is one of my favourite spices, not only for its aniseed flavour but also for its natural healing powers. It is useful for nausea, digestion, bloating, stomach cramps, poor appetite and—something to remember after childbirth—this tea is a fabulous cure for a hangover.

1 tsp fennel seeds

Infuse in a mug of boiling water for 3–5 minutes.

warm spiced milk

A mug of warm milk before bedtime is an effective nighttime sedative. When spices are added, you have a wonderful digestive tonic as well. Sweet dreams.

1 mug low-fat milk

1 tsp mixed spice or cinnamon

Gently warm milk and spices in a small saucepan over a low heat, stirring regularly. Alternatively, heat in the microwave for 60 seconds. Stir well.

Hot Choc-cinnamon

Here is a hot chocolate drink that is nourishing. Cocoa is iron-rich and cinnamon assists digestion, nausea and circulation and maintains blood sugar levels. Add a small dash of manuka honey for antibacterial properties.

1 mug low-fat milk

1 tsp cocoa

1 tsp cinnamon

Gently warm milk in a small saucepan over a low heat, stirring regularly. Add cocoa and cinnamon and stir until combined. Alternatively, heat in the microwave.

Part Three

when baby makes two

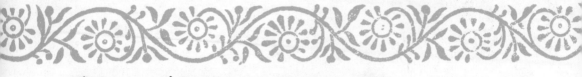

✿ Breastfeeding and Beyond

Time is limited when caring for a newborn and it is easy to neglect your own health. A well-balanced diet is essential post-birth for physical recovery and to maintain much needed energy levels. Ready-made, home-cooked meals will ensure you consume all of your essential nutrients. Suggested recipes are listed in the section entitled Breastfeeding and Beyond. Sleepless nights, recovering from childbirth, a newborn baby—the demands on a new mother are enormous. However, this is a very special phase of life and should be enjoyed rather than witnessed through a fog of fatigue.

Maintaining good health is as important post-partum as it was during pregnancy. A woman's body works harder during pregnancy than at any other time of her life. We have discussed the nutritional demands and the physical are more than obvious. Reward and refuel your body with wholesome foods. These will aid physical recovery, manage emotions and provide much needed energy. As in pregnancy, eat regularly to maintain blood sugar levels, sustain energy and avoid fatigue.

Time is going to be your greatest restraint as you settle into feeding and caring routines. Meals that have been pre-cooked and frozen will be an absolute blessing. If you did not manage to prepare meals prior to birth, enlist family and friends to do it for you now. You will find a list of recipes suitable for freezing and post-partum at the end of this chapter.

Breastfeeding

Substantial worldwide research shows there are considerable nutritional and health benefits from breastfeeding. Breast milk is the most complete and perfect food for a baby for the first six months of its life. It meets all nutritional needs and provides antibodies that protect against infections and disease.

Breast milk is rich in protein and carbohydrates for growth and energy, essential fatty acids for continued brain development and calcium for healthy teeth and bones. It also has a high fluid content to hydrate your baby.

Breast milk changes according to the needs of your growing baby throughout the first six months of breastfeeding. It also changes during a feed, from a watery texture to a thicker, creamier texture containing more fat. This allows the baby to quench its thirst first, then satisfy its hunger. The change in milk also introduces the baby to different tastes and textures, making the infant more inclined to try new foods as it matures.

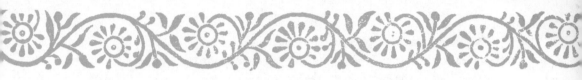

Colostrum is produced during pregnancy and is very rich in protein. It is present in high concentrations in the first few days of lactation and then mixes in with breast milk for the first month or so. Its function is to develop the immune system and the bowel. It coats the gut, produces healthy gut bacteria and then promotes and removes the first stool. In other words, it gets the bowel moving. This is a very important and final stage of bowel development.

Breastfeeding is a very personal decision and for some women the choice is not their own. Inadequate supplies or other complications can arise, but the first few important feeds are usually achievable. If you do decide to breastfeed, there are many benefits.

Benefits to mother:

- significantly reduces the risk of breast and ovarian cancer and osteoporosis
- encourages pregnancy weight loss as fat stores are used for breastfeeding
- assists in postnatal recovery by producing hormones that help to repair the uterus
- minimises chances of developing postnatal depression
- encourages mother/baby bonding
- fewer nappies to change as there is no waste product in breast milk.

Benefits to baby:

- meets *all* nutritional requirements
- easy to digest, with nutrients more effectively absorbed (especially iron)
- contains antibodies to protect against infection
- develops the bowel
- rich in essential fatty acids for continued brain development
- less likely to develop diarrhoea and respiratory infections, as well as diabetes, allergies and obesity later in life.

There is evidence that breast-fed babies are more likely to develop healthy eating patterns. Breast-fed babies instinctively learn to control their own food intake. When they are satisfied, they stop suckling. Bottle-fed babies are often forced to finish the bottle, whether hungry or not. It has been claimed that this can develop overeating habits that carry through into both childhood and adulthood.

Breastfeeding can be a challenging and sometimes painful experience for mothers. Sore, tender breasts, cracked nipples and mastitis are the more unattractive virtues of learning to breastfeed. The following remedies may assist:

- eating garlic—fabulous for mastitis
- increase intake of B-complex vitamins—B6 is great for sore breasts and mastitis and sources include wholegrains, wheatgerm, green leafy vegetables and lean meat
- foods high in zinc and vitamin C and E, in addition to fresh air and applying breast milk are the best remedies to promote healing of early nipple damage
- cabbage compresses wrapped around the breast are a great way of soothing over-full and tender breasts.

A healthy diet is as important during lactation as it was during pregnancy. There is no need to avoid any specific foods unless your baby is reacting to them, or if you or the father have identified food allergies. Monitor your baby's response to different foods you eat and judge for yourself. Flavours are transferred to breast milk, but if your baby can tolerate a spicy stir-fry, go ahead and enjoy. In fact it is beneficial to expose your baby to a variety of tastes and flavours. It can lessen the chance of rearing a fussy eater.

You, your breast milk and your baby will benefit if your diet is rich in the following nutrients:

- calcium and magnesium—for continued development of teeth and bones and protection against osteoporosis. Continue eating 4 servings daily (5 for vegetarians)
- essential fatty acids—a baby's brain is not fully developed at birth, so keep up the omega 3
- vitamin C—daily servings are important as neither you nor your baby can store this nutrient
- vitamin E
- B-group vitamins (especially B12)
- zinc
- protein
- carbohydrates.

It is imperative *not* to diet when breastfeeding, despite any urgency you may feel to get back into prenatal shape. Fat stores were specifically accumulated during pregnancy to be converted to breast milk. These stores will be used up and you will naturally lose any excess weight. Strict dieting will deplete the quantity of breast milk, which can deny your baby of complete nutrition. You will also become fatigued very quickly. Energy must be sourced from a nourishing diet and as breast milk is almost 90% water, it is vital to drink *at least* eight glasses of water per day.

Blender drinks such as smoothies, milkshakes, frappes and fruit and vegetable juices are ideal meals for lactating mothers. Time and energy are scarce, so the ease and convenience of a complete meal in one cup is very appealing. My *Berry Blast* is made in minutes and contains protein, calcium, vitamin C, zinc, omega 3 and antioxidants.

Soups are perfect as you can make large quantities and freeze individual portions for those days when you are too tired or busy to cook. You will find this beneficial during the first few months of motherhood. Soups are great during lactation as their high water content keeps you and your breastmilk hydrated.

All you need to make a delicious soup is a large, heavy-based pot and good quality stock, preferably homemade. Stock is the base of your soup and a good protein source. If purchasing stock, always buy salt-reduced and read the labels for added preservatives. Good quality organic stocks are available from health food stores, delis and gourmet grocery stores.

253

Beyond (post-partum)

Whether you choose to breastfeed or not, your body still requires specific nutrients to recover and recharge. Protein, carbohydrates, essential fatty acids, iron, calcium and vitamin C are the ones to watch.

Fatigue, anaemia and constipation are common complaints after childbirth. Fatigue is usually the result of lack of sleep. Maintain energy by eating regularly and choosing healthy, low GI foods and recipes. Fatigue can also be an indication of anaemia. A substantial amount of blood is lost during childbirth, which the body does prepare for during pregnancy. Some women may lose more blood, which may result in a low red blood cell count. Maintain a high intake of iron-rich foods (see Iron). Consult your health practitioner if feeling continually tired or if you appear paler than usual.

Constipation often worsens during the first few days after delivery. It is also normal to have a sore bottom following labour. Add to this the possibility of stitches, and the thought of your first post-birth bowel movement can be terrifying. Dietary fibre and lots of fluids should get things moving. See Constipation for food sources, remedies and recipes. The Banana and Prune Smoothie, Mixed grain natural muesli and Spicy Lentil Soup are effective options.

recipes for post-partum

The following are recipes that can be pre-prepared and frozen for up to two months for later use:

Tasty Tuna Patties

Mini Salmon Quiches

Slow-cooked Beef and Vegetable Stew

Soups—all

Muffins—all

Marinated uncooked meats in freezer bags

Brazil Nut Burgers

Chickpea and Vegetable Curry

Healthy Breakfast Loaf

Fruit Creams

Chunky Pesto Spread

Hummus

Your need for energy in the form of complex carbohydrates and low GI foods is enormous during lactation. Try:

Nourishing Nut and Seed Mix

Fruit and Nut Bars

Leek and Mushroom Frittata

Ginger Salmon Curry

Tuna Pastas

Salmon and Egg Salad

Mixed Grain Porridge

Mixed Grain Natural Muesli

Tropical C Fruit Salad

Fruit Salad with the Works

Steamed Chicken in a Delicate Ginger and
   Lemon Broth

Quinoa Capsicum Treats

Beef Pasta with Almond and Avocado Pesto

Steak Sandwich with Tomato Salsa

Chicken Mango Salad

Stuffed Mushrooms (with or without
   steak)

Roasted Lamb with Spinach, Almonds and
   Prunes

The following recipes are made in minutes and provide a huge nutritional boost:

Bara-Burger with Babaganoush

Rosemary Lamb and Tomato Bake

Boiled Eggs with Vegemite Soldiers

Egg Pesto (pesto pre-made and frozen)

Tuna, Leek and Mushroom Sauté

Tuna Pastas

Sardines on Toast

Mediterranean Lamb Pizzas or
   Vegetarian Pita Pizzas

Blender Drinks—all

Grilled Vegetable Skewers with Hummus
   (hummus pre-made and frozen)

Grilled Figs with Cinnamon

special Thanks

This book would never have been possible without the support and enthusiasm of my wonderful family and friends.

First and foremost to Paul, whose unwavering belief, support and encouragement got me through all the bumps, motivated me to 'get back into the kitchen', put 'us' on hold for over two years, and whose humane generosity and love has scarred my heart in the most beautiful way.

To our gorgeous Charlie who brings an indescribable amount of love and laughter into our lives and was always most appreciative of a failed recipe.

To my wonderful mother and my aunts for their unwavering belief and love.

To Katrina, my angel in disguise. Her encouragement, guidance, kindness and pregnancy of her own must be accredited to the birth of *Feeding the Bump*.

To my recipe and taste testers, especially Clare, Janna, Christy, Linda and again Katrina, thank you so much for taking the time to test the dishes and for the helpful feedback.

To James Valentine, my mentor in so many ways.

To my publishing team at Allen & Unwin who have made a dream come true, particularly to Jo Paul and Catherine Milne who believed in the *Bump* from the very beginning. And to Joanne Holliman for weaving her magic through my words, turning a manuscript into a masterpiece, and for her unwavering patience.
Thank you all.

And finally, to all mothers, expecting mothers and future mothers. Bearing a child is such an amazing and blessed experience. I hope that *Feeding the Bump* can enrich that experience and guide you through a happy, comfortable pregnancy and deliver you a beautiful, healthy baby.

Resources

Conception, Pregnancy and Birth, Dr Miriam Stoppard
Food is Medicine, Pierre-Jean Cousin
Low GI Food, Dr Susanna Holt
New Pregnancy and Birth Book, Dr Miriam Stoppard
Nutrition for Life, Lisa Hark and Darwin Deen
Nutrition for Life, Catherine Saxelby
Simply Healthy, Sally James
Spice Notes, Ian Hemphill
The Cook's Companion, Stephanie Alexander
The Natural Way to a Better Pregnancy, Francesca Naish and Janette Roberts
Up the Duff, Kaz Cooke
What to Eat When You're Expecting, Arlene Eisenberg, Heidi Murkoff and Sandee Hathaway
What to Expect When You're Expecting, Arlene Eisenberg, Heidi Murkoff and Sandee Hathaway
Your Over–35 Week-by-Week Pregnancy Guide, M. Kelly Shanahan

Dairy Australia
Department of Nutrition and Dietetics, Royal Prince Alfred Hospital
Food Standards Australia and New Zealand
NSW Food Authority
NSW Department of Health
Nutrition Australia
Women's Health Institute, Royal Hospital for Women

www.foodauthority.nsw.gov.au
www.foodstandards.gov.au
www.nal.usda.gov

Index